Minding Your Matter

Dear Sis & Jim;
I hope you kick back &
enjoy reading my new book —
then take a "walk."
It was great talking to you two;
so let's keep doing it!
Take good care of yourselves
& each other —
Always,
[signature] & Carol

Minding Your Matter

A Breakthrough Health and Fitness Model Without Formal Diets and Exercises

Dr. Larry Wonderling, Ph.D.

Cape Foundation Publications
San Francisco, California

Cape Foundation Publications
San Francisco, California
Email: capfound@aol.com.

First printed 2005

ISBN: 0-9659415-7-4

LCCN: 2005929987

Printed and bound in the United States of America.
Cover Design by Norman Cyr
Editor: Carol Eversole

CONTENTS

FOREWORD xiii

PROLOGUE xvii

PART I: Know Your Enemies to Health and Fitness

Chapter 1: Never Cross the Street With Your Eyes Closed 3

Chapter 2: The Uneven Starting Line 11

Chapter 3: Medical Double-Speak 18

Chapter 4: Education's Misguided Priorities 26

Chapter 5: Make Sure Your Friends Really Are 33

PART II: Know Yourself and How You Affect Your Health and Fitness

Chapter 6: What Are You? 43

Chapter 7: You Are What You Eat 48

Chapter 8: You Are What You Do 62

Chapter 9: What Matters Is You 77

Chapter 10: Mind Your Own Business 87

PART III: Know the Best Health and Fitness Strategy for You

Chapter 11: Health and Fitness Options 101

Chapter 12: Get Ready To Go For It 106

Chapter 13: The Exercise Road to Fitness is a Footpath. 113

Chapter 14: If Your Menu's Getting all Greasy, Toss It 147

Chapter 15: And the Winner is… 158

APPENDIX

A. Body Mass Index Chart 163

B. BMI Formula using Meters and Kilograms 164

C. Blood Pressure Basics 164

D. Pulse Basics 165

E. Type of Calories Per Gram 165

F.	Calorie Burning Activity Chart	165
G.	Stress Questionnaire	165
H.	Cholesterol Facts	167
I.	Obesity Facts and References	167
J.	Activity Facts and References	169
K.	Body Composition	170
L.	Body Composition Standards	170
M.	New Food Pyramid	171
N.	Solution to Child's Puzzle	171

LIST OF PHOTOGRAPHS 172

BIBLIOGRAPHY 173

INDEX 177

ABOUT THE AUTHOR 181

Dedication

To all my friends, flabby or firm, who inspired the writing of this book.

Acknowledgements

No matter how many books I write, shaping ideas into a readable manuscript doesn't seem to work without the help of friends, colleagues and those neighbors I barely know. Even then I rediscover I'm not finished. I'm still not confident it's any good. So a final tweaking of the final draft is vital before the manuscript is indelibly transformed into a book for all to view. To John Burton, Lynn and John Drocco, Jan Elster, Linda and Bob Hanna, Shirley Kennedy, Bob St.Claire and Vicky Walker I deeply appreciate your feedback and encouragement. To Ben Levy for his help in formatting. To my dear friend and primary editor, Carol Eversole, your hard work always overwhelms me.

MINDING YOUR MATTER

FOREWORD

By Professor Bob Lualhati

In retrospect, my life has clearly been devoted to earnest participation in and observation of all that's significant in my environment. As an athlete, I have managed to regularly care for my body since my first teenage sports competition. As an educator, I have watched in deep frustration students' and faculty's gradual loss of interest in Physical Education, despite my efforts to reverse the negative trend.

I chose teaching, knowing that young people's values are powerfully influenced by their mentors. What I hadn't factored into my decision was education's possible negative influences on the young.

In academia, Physical Education has historically been a low priority, and with budget cuts, P.E. programs have usually been the first to go. Unfortunately, the message to most tractable students has been that fitness isn't all that important. In fact the true objective of all education is to prepare students physically, as well as intellectually. An ancient Roman satirist once said, "a sound mind in a sound body." This is what is called a "Total Education." Any educational system falls short of meeting its obligation to its various students by offering less.

Because of this, I have watched students grow fatter and softer within an educational system that has done less and less to reward or even encourage student participation in sports or exercise programs.

To verify my concerns, I introduced a Fitness Education Program regarding the physical fitness and exercise attitudes of incoming and outgoing students. That was twenty-one years ago. This study within our P.E. Department at Skyline College has regretfully documented the relentless physical deterioration of students with alarming loss of muscle strength and excesses in fat weight. These findings are based on the demographics of both young women and men, and by 1989 the trend and its interpretation were shockingly clear. College students were becoming increasing overweight and disinterested in exercise or fitness.

As of 2005 the trend continues, and our nation is finally acknowledging the gravity of the obesity problem that is no less of an epidemic than AIDS or smoking.

My good friend, Dr. Larry Wonderling, and I have shared these conclusions for decades. Invariably during social gatherings, the deplorable physical condition of our youth and senior citizens ends up the main topic of conversation.

We agreed years ago that obesity is infecting both genders of all ages and socioeconomic situations. We both knew years ago that no one is immune to obesity or the diseases caused by such excessive weight and poor fitness. Obesity does not discriminate. Both genders, all ethnic and age groups are paying dearly for their sedentary lifestyles!

I have long been a strident opponent of quick fix diets, diet pills and short-term exercise programs. So has Dr. Wonderling. We further recognized that the only effective treatment or prevention of obesity is a change from a sedentary lifestyle to a physically active one, regardless of age. We also knew too well the obstacles in modern day societies that block good fitness and health habits. Another book needed writing.

I am delighted to have collaborated with my friend in the completion of this long overdue, one of a kind, fitness and health book. Refreshingly, the book is clear and objective in exposing all social, as well as physical obstacles to permanent fitness. I also strongly endorse all of the exercises and eating recommendations. They are founded in research and empirical conclusions by many health and fitness experts.

The major premise inherent in this book is that healthful lifestyle changes are unlikely unless the exercises and eating recommendations blend easily with ones daily activities. *Minding Your Matter* promotes no apparatus, gadgets, pills or special diets that separate the regimen from one's daily life. In consultation with Larry, we both made certain our health and fitness plan was a seamless blend with anyone's life and suitable for any age. We have both used such a plan of healthy activities and sensible eating during most of our own lives. We both know how well it works, and all it requires is willingness to change, taking charge of one's body and common sense.

Professor Bob Lualhati

PROLOGUE

The next time you stand before a full-length mirror, take a good look. Whether it's a satisfying or embarrassing sight, keep looking and not just at those acceptable parts. What you see is a reflection of the most precious of all miracles—human life. Usually when we think of miracles, we envision sight for the blind, redemption, parting seas or resurrection. Yet, how we simply take that miraculous image in the mirror for granted is a fathomless puzzle. So take a closer look. From head to toe, every bit is you; the most astonishing and underrated of all miracles.

You are a breathing, thinking, remarkable phenomenon. What you're looking at is so outrageously complex, it can be examined, but never understood. You are looking at a self-contained energy system incased in an exquisite network of tissue, billions of cells, neurons and chemicals. It is indeed a living universe, capable of preserving or neglecting our planet. Such an awesome creation is hardly an accident, yet no one really knows how each of us originally got here. This may be life's most baffling mystery—a miraculous whole far greater than the sum of all of its parts, yet it can be reduced to nearly two-thirds water and a dozen or so chemicals, all once valued at about $1.98.

Your mirror provides only a glimpse of the mysterious miracle of miracles, and caring for this astonishing presence is your most vital responsibility. Be ever aware that only you have supreme power over your own universe of mind and matter. It awaits your orders, which are capable of hurting or healing yourself.

This is the message embedded in this book. Don't you dare take the miracle—yourself—for granted! The power of our miracle over all other creatures belies just how vulnerable each of us really is. There are countless adversaries out there to harm us—from viruses no bigger than a fragmented thought, to the enormous size and thunder of attacking armies. The most insidious of all those enemies, however, is our own abuse of the miracle. It's simply up to each of us to take care of ourselves—to take care of our own mind and matter from this point on.

Improving your health clearly begins by simply monitoring how you look and feel. Amazingly, just gazing at your body tells you a lot about your health and wellness. Then, learning what you can do to improve what you see depends on understanding what factors shape the state of your health. Finally, you need to establish ways of permanently improving your health and physical fitness. Embracing these initial steps to better health is easier than you think. Just taking a few moments once a week to check how you look and feel is a *great start*.

There are a variety of symptoms that provide solid hints about your health. A constant red face, even when not embarrassed, suggests high blood pressure; chest pains could announce heart problems or indigestion; pallid skin may signal anemia or oxygen deprivation; and scab-like lesions that won't go away could spell skin cancer. In fact, any abrupt, unfamiliar or unexpected change in how you look or feel is always especially noteworthy.

Yet, these potentially alarming symptoms can all be too subtle to notice. There is, however, another more obvious visual symptom that, ironically, is too often overlooked. It's called *adipose tissue*, or the more familiar term, *fat*. In fact, fat is the clearest, most observable reminder about the state of our health, especially when fat becomes excessive.

Too much fat is obesity, the final assault of fat on our bodies. It's a condition so visibly obvious, it not only severely burdens our health, it may cruelly blemish our self-confidence. Obesity is hard to ignore as people side step our girth in narrow corridors, avoid the seat adjoining our hips on planes or snicker and point as we waddle by.

Since appearance is all too frequently worshiped in our society, fat is arguably the most measurable and recognizable symptom of our mental and physical well being. In this book, these are all good reasons why fat serves as a constant barometer forecasting the state of our health and physical fitness. It's an inverse relationship, or simply put, as our weight barometer goes up, our health and fitness go down.

These easily observable and well-researched findings make unarguable sense. Yet, why is obesity such a pandemic problem? Certainly, the most tenable answer is a troubling paradox as well: too many of us get so used to being pudgy, stout, chubby or just plain fat we tend to overlook, deny or even reason away its damaging existence. We take the obvious excessive weight for granted or righteously sneer at those who snicker.

ꕤ ꕤ

All of the above underscores the major purpose of this book: *to increase awareness of yourself and all of the obstacles undermining your health and fitness, while guiding you toward a more fulfilling, healthful lifestyle.*

Our strategy will also move you away from the industry of dieting and those athletic club physical fitness programs with their high relapse rates. Following the teachings in this book won't cost you the frustrations or expense of special diets and grueling exercise regimens. You will just look and feel better than ever. That's a promise.

Part I

Know Your Enemies to Health and Fitness

CHAPTER 1

Never Cross the Street with Your Eyes Closed

Resist the above warning of the all too obvious and you'll end up in really poor health or no health—that's another promise. It's sort of Russian roulette with cars, one of the more obvious adversaries out there that keep trying to nail you—in more ways than you think!

But, you may argue, motor vehicles aren't the threat they once were. They've been around for a century and we're used to them. Besides, there are crosswalks, traffic signals, open eyes, fancy footwork and our flawless sophistication in coping with urban hazards. We are so accustomed to traffic; the relentless proliferation of cars is no longer a menace.

Oh? Then why do thousands of pedestrians and drivers get killed or maimed yearly by motor vehicles? And, why is our extreme dependence on motor vehicles also unwittingly contributing to our nation's obesity? It's because we are so used to them, our sense of safety is *blind.*

This may well be the major theme of Part I. We get so inured to comfort, inactivity and so many other threats to our bodies, we tend to take urban hazards for *granted*—we simply lose *sight* of them. Like the white noise of TV static between working channels, let it crackle long enough and we no longer hear it. As pedestrians, automobiles can still break our legs in the crosswalks, and as drivers, weaken our legs by disuse.

That's why this book, unlike most books on health and fitness, begins at the beginning instead of somewhere in the middle. In other words, in order to get fit and healthy, you first need to be reminded of all those dangerous enemies to your health. They are so taken for granted they've become stealth bombers that strike without warning.

Living, especially in urban society, is a taunting array of contradictions. We believe we're the safest, healthiest country ever, while losing sight of our struggle against countless urban obstacles. It's a war, and should we surrender to our indifference, which most of us do, we'll be invaded by a variety of good reasons for poor health.

Getting thoroughly reacquainted with all those dangerously subtle urban adversaries to good health and fitness is the major goal of Part I. After all, how can we possibly challenge environmental enemies to good health unless we know what they are? Informed decisions about what's good for our health and fitness come from an awareness we can easily lose in taking everything for *granted*—by closing our eyes.

☙ ❧

Third Millennium Americans are citizens of the most powerful nation in the world. We've become world leaders in everything, especially consumerism. We buy enough clothes yearly to easily supply the entire world with our hand-me-downs. We buy so many cars per family that most cities double as parking lots. We burn more fuel to operate our private vehicles than most of the world uses to operate their nations. We are consummate shoppers, rarely in search of necessities.

These comments, however, aren't "tongue in cheek" hyperbole, so try to restrain the smile. It's the sobering economic paradox of our fiscal prosperity. *Our country can only continue to flourish if we keep buying what we don't really need.* So, clutching one of our credit cards, we patriotically engage in one of our favorite mindless obligations—buying *stuff* we don't really need.

An enormous amount of that unnecessary *stuff* has something to do with *food*, perhaps our most cherished obsession. The typical upper middle class family of three has a kitchen of restaurant magnitude, with two dozen skillets, pots and pans; three cupboards of plates, glasses and other food containers, and a minimum of eighteen drawers for the hundred fifty utensils, including knifes, silverware, dicers, mashers, slicers, crushers, strainers, pounders, ad infinitum! We never have enough *things* to prepare our food and, of course, our kitchens are never big enough. Even our bookshelf has more cookbooks than a small library; and along with professional athletes, chefs are some of our biggest heroes.

Having said all of that with a "little" tongue in cheek, it's still apparent that eating in the United States is more than a basic biological need or physiological process. It's a sacred ritual, a cultural obsession, a gluttonous compulsion. The bottom line is the sad, scientific fact that we eat too much; which is a psychological phenomenon, as well as a biological curse. It's been embedded in our psyche since infancy that three squares a day are essential to good health and a sound social adjustment.

After all, we were well trained to eat at least three hearty meals a day by our parents, who learned from their parents, who learned as well from their parents—you know those pioneers who physically and strenuously worked in the fields *fifteen hours a day*. Well, we still insist on our daily three meals, even though the overwhelming majority of us may have physically strenuous work that amounts to *ten minutes a day*.

After a half day of work or play, that Pavlovian noon whistle announces time to eat again. Our watch or the wall clock tells us we need nourishment and out comes the brown bag or the necessary trip to the nearest restaurant. In a hurry? The cafeteria or fast food line will do.

As well trained, obedient adults, we know noon means hunger, even when we're not hungry. It doesn't really matter anymore. For most of us, eating is no longer associated with survival. The tradition, with its eating ritual, is all that matters. Look around, because everyone else is doing it. Maybe it's a peer pressure thing. More likely we are so adaptable, we've lost awareness of our choices. The reason hardly matters anymore.

We are hooked and we've become a nation of lumpos. We're over the 50% mark for corpulence in the U.S.A. We are number one in the world for excessive adipose tissue. People, the very foundation of our nation, are slowing down to a waddle with too much fat—and they're getting fatter!

In lieu of vomitoriums, crash diets, starvation, surgical stomach reduction and "uppers," people may have to begin using more of their physiology than just their digestive system. They may have to rediscover how food is processed once it enters their mouth, why the human body has about 656 skeletal muscles, and why Darwin's Natural Selection may be greatly reducing this number of muscles through disuse.

Food is just one of an endless assortment of potentially sinister obstacles to good health. We eat all the time because we need food to survive. At least that's what's been jammed down our overworked throats since our first mouthful of rich, creamy milk from mother's breast. Now, we're so used to eating, we rarely ask ourselves about amount or nutrition. We're just habitual eaters whether we need it or not. Need is irrelevant. Lunch is an absolute necessity—why? Because it is!

Food isn't our only potential enemy. Living in industrial societies spawns all kinds of health adversaries and they are often difficult to spot, let alone judge. The smoke and mirrors of marketing tend to obscure the good from the not so good, which makes urban living more treacherous than we think.

If it's marketed, it's user friendly, even when it isn't. While preaching the good life, marketers also teach poor fitness through atrophy. These marketers intimate that *use it or lose it*, is an old mythical grandma-ism. Science, however, agrees with grandma. The less physically active we are the fatter and softer we become as our muscles waste away. Remember when you got that cast off your arm or leg? What a flabby mess until you started reusing it.

Look around. There are enemies to our health and fitness lurking everywhere. So, back to those big, comfortable cars with the six speaker CD players, deep, cushy seats and soothing temperature control. They easily morph into a living room where we're constantly encouraged to kick back, relax and rest those legs we rarely use. As we look around, we may also notice that cars—big cars—are as prevalent as lunch. Yet neither is vital to our survival.

Another indispensable part of our urban struggle is television. Sets come in all sizes and shapes with the same anti-activity, spectator pitch. It's a compelling sell that has seduced most of the nation. We're invited to rest our bodies and minds as long as we want, and it doesn't cost us a single calorie.

The Third Millennium technology offers countless additional ways to discourage activity. There are computers, video games galore, cell phones, all sorts of chairs, seats and desk jobs with more chairs and seats. What a sluggish life we've become accustomed to.

Like medications, the marvels of science and technology can help us or harm us, and the difference between help and harm becomes increasingly blurred as we adapt too easily to comfort and convenience. Marketing and tradition have an uncanny way of rearranging our health and fitness priorities until what *feels* good to us finally trumps what's *actually* good for us. That's when we can't see those proverbial trees for the forest.

Then it's time to detach yourself from the urban marketing hustle long enough to clarify your thinking, reexamine the positive and negative aspects of convenience oriented living and make some informed choices.

That's what this chapter is all about. As your eyes open wide in heightened awareness of the health and fitness obstacles in your way, you'll be more than capable of doing something about them.

Did you know that any worthwhile nonfiction book has a definite message of some kind in every chapter? This health and fitness book is no different. Usually each chapter in health books—or any nonfiction book for that matter—contains about two paragraphs of important researched or empirically established ideas. Those ideas represent the most critical information for the reader to understand. Yet, too frequently, in an author's zeal to transform a pamphlet of information into a thick book, the treasure of ideas is lost in a morass of redundant babble. These are the health books with twenty-page chapters that are really providing only three real worthwhile facts, (researched information) with the remainder of the words being just pure prosey glitz.

Unfortunately, once we choose to write a health book rather than a hand-out, we authors have made our choice of writing lots of words to say very little. Even those painstakingly detailed texts written for information hungry students are generally too long and ponderous.

Now that you know why many big books are so wordy and hard to understand, you'll be pleased to note that each chapter in this book will conclude with those obscured facts clearly outlined, pamphlet style. Read the research-based *Fact Summary* over and over, because it's the message you really need to understand.

Fact Summary:

1. Since your body is a genuine miracle and the only one you've got, don't take it for granted.
2. Keep your eyes open. You can't defend against obstacles to good health unless you know what they are.

3. Most of us eat too much and exercise too little.
4. The urban life of stressors, excessive conveniences, inactivity and overindulgences is trying to kill us.
5. Regain your human potential. Think for yourself with informed choices.

CHAPTER 2

The Uneven Starting Line

The title of this chapter says it all and what it says is not fair. Some people seem to be born with a warehouse of advantages while others begin life with barely enough potential to fill a shoebox. That's the tragic inequity of the human miracle.

We have architects from within that establish, in general terms, our anatomical, neurobiochemical and psychological predisposition for success, good health and longevity. It's an incredible part of creation, except that the starting line is anything but straight. It's as deep as it is wide, with most of us so far behind the front-runners it's hardly a contest.

Sorry! The miracle of human life simply doesn't start with equal opportunities, especially in urban societies. A quick scan of any crowded street is all the evidence we need. As a species we're so similar, other species probably can't tell us apart. Yet, from our human vantage point, the differences are astounding. We're tall, short, ugly, pretty, clumsy, agile, well-formed or deformed, etc. These physical characteristics are called *phenotypes* and help establish our status in society. The tall, broad-shouldered, handsome male and the petite, beautiful female will be clearly advantaged in urban societies that initially define us by our appearance. The miraculous mystery underlying these socially unfair differences is our individual *genotype*—our genes—the most basic unit of heredity.

Each genetic code represents a curse or blessing to the individual well beyond those obvious physical characteristics. Our basic mental processes as well, including intelligence, are nestled within our cellular structure at birth. Our disease propensity, pain tolerance, mathematical, musical and athletic abilities have genetic links. You name it, and good or bad, genes have plenty to do with it. You might even argue—what we become or fail to be is not our fault. That debate could fill another book.

☙ ❧

Fortunately, to round out our magnificent organizational design, there are a few other factors that help or hinder physical and social prosperity in life. Loving, bright, stable, supportive parents will certainly nurture and help maximize the best of one's genetic possibilities. Luck and one's environment also has a lot to do with how our gene pool cares for us. This chapter, however, is about how one's struggle on the outside affects those thousands of genetic critters on the inside, with their potential to help or hinder us.

There's another inside variable that may play the most important role in getting the most out of our genes. It's called *volition*. A bit difficult to define, volition has something to do with will power, determination, motivation, tenacity and no doubt faith. It's probably also closely related to resilience, courage and optimism. Operationally it means doing more than your best in any situation—giving that proverbial one hundred ten percent even if your achievement is only average.

Whether it originates somewhere in your gene pool, like intelligence, is clearly debatable.

More importantly, volition does exist and provides assurances that we can effectively challenge most any obstacle—including genetic ones—if we try hard enough. It's not our fault if we got short-changed genetically, but within our predetermined limitations, there's plenty of room for improvement.

☙ ❧

Obesity is a vital and excellent example of those inner genetic catalysts to health and fitness. What better example of genes at work than massive bodies of fleshy, jiggling flab that are so hard to pass by unnoticed.

Obesity is an overwhelmingly obvious, bigger than life symptom of a health disaster in progress. It's the big screaming announcement to the whole community of onlookers that this person is headed for pain, disease and early death. Just a few statistics should be enough to convince anyone that obesity is a world class killer.

How about the American Cancer Society's comprehensive study since 1982, its conclusions are staggering. As we become noticeably overweight, our risk of cancer begins to increase as well, by fifty to sixty percent. Types of cancers include esophagus, colon, liver, breasts, cervix and prostate. The Center for Disease Control (CDC) has some alarming statistics of its own. The 1980 fifteen percent obesity rate increased to twenty-seven percent in 1999, and it's still climbing. The CDC further reports obesity as "central to the development of many chronic diseases such as Type Two Diabetes, heart disease, hypertension and cancer."

George W. Bush's Health and Human Services Secretary, Tommy Thompson, added to the alarm in

July 2003 when he said sixty-five percent of Americans are overweight. As alarming, Surgeon General Richard Carmona reported that nearly nine million kids are seriously overweight.

Before your eyelids begin their fluttering heaviness with the drone of statistics, try to stay awake for just a few more numbers. Another 2003 study finds that if we all reduced to normal weight in the United States, ninety thousand lives would be spared. Hang on! Just one more stat: In 2000, just one year, the total cost of obesity in the United States was estimated at $117 billion; $61 billion for direct medical costs and $56 billion for medically related costs.

Clearly the rate of obesity is a matter of major public health concern. With obesity continuing to increase in the United States, CDC's 2004 warnings are even more strident, "Our worst fears were confirmed…it's going to overtake tobacco…obesity has to be job number one for us in terms of chronic disease." An even more recent update appears in the May 2004 *MONITOR*, an American Psychological Association publication. The article quotes a congressional report based on research literature that states, "Studies are beginning to show that obesity is a bigger health threat than smoking and alcohol abuse, and it leads to increase of chronic diseases such as diabetes, heart disease, stroke and cancer…studies provide strong evidence that prevention efforts focusing on diet, exercise and other lifestyle changes can substantially reduce these health risks in high risk groups." There are an abundance of other overweight studies with warnings and the same grim prophecy. In the Appendix under I, there's a summary of these studies (obesity facts).

If you don't mind sabotaging quality and length of life, keep putting on the pounds. And that's a consensual fact even without the numbers. Just look around your neighborhood.

One more caveat you've probably heard many times. The earlier disease symptoms are detected, the greater the cure rate when treated. Clear enough? Everybody knows that. Yet, how is it that fat, the most noticeable, glaringly obvious symptom in the whole world of symptoms is routinely overlooked? Certainly not because it's too tiny to see. That question is answered in another chapter; which is one more reason to keep reading.

Back to genetics and those inner critters that ordain what each of us will be. Well, not quite. You might as well stop placing all the blame for your bulging love handles on genes alone. If your eyes are steel blue or mushy gray, height short or tall, feet huge or tiny, and nose pugged, it's really not your fault. And you might as well appreciate those physical features. They're your personal, individual signature. In fact, you'll be surprised how much more others will like your appearance if you do. Anyway, there's not much you can do about it *naturally*, no matter how hard you try. Yeah, we know. There are color contact lenses, shoe lifts, plastic surgery, etc., and if that's your strategy, you may not be particularly interested in what this book has to say.

☙ ❧

Excess weight, however, is not an immutable mass encased in granite. It's a malleable systemic condition partially regulated by genes, and profoundly obedient to your habits.

Granted, understanding the complexities of bio-chemical programming going on deep in your cells wouldn't do a thing to improve your health or fitness. It's also highly likely that all you may be interested in knowing is what you already know. But just in case you have zero understanding of the genome, here are the very basics—all you need to know.

Each one of us has a somewhat different energy metabolism that's kind of like a thermostat genetically regulating our weight. Low metabolism people are slow caloric burners. They get fat easier. Those with high metabolism are blast furnaces. They tend to stay thin with minimal effort.

Hunger and appetite hormones are other biochemical contributors to weight gains and losses. If your common sense response to all this is, "so what, since there's nothing I can do about individual genotypes," please don't despair. What all those basics actually mean is that, if everyone's weight related activities were identical, we'd all be stuck with whatever body mass our genes prescribed. Of course, we all behave differently, which means we can individually alter our weight.

My favorite example of overcoming genetic boundaries is *me* and that invisible force called *volition*. My genetically programmed intelligence, as measured by standardized tests, is an Intelligence Quotient (IQ) of about 98, or very average. Average IQ's will assure us a high school diploma and a community college degree with average effort. Graduating from a four year college or university with an average IQ will be tougher, requiring extra effort; while a Master's Degree would be even more demanding. Well, possessing my average IQ gene, I managed a not too surprising "C" average Bachelor's Degree, "B" average Master's and a straight "A" Ph.D. Degree. No, I didn't get a gene transplant; I just *really, really* wanted those advanced degrees.

While those other graduate students, with their 130 plus IQ genes, studied three hours a night, I'll bet you know what I was up to. I beat those genetic studs by studying six or seven hours a day—every day. Was it worth it? Sure was! I *really, really* wanted those advanced degrees. That is the key to poking the upper limits of many of our genetic ceilings—volition, aka motivation, drive, determination.

Similar to IQ genes, the overwhelming majority of weight genes permit alterations in your fat size. If you have a sluggish metabolism comparable to an IQ of 73, you may never be a Bantamweight boxer or a slim line model, but there's plenty of room for improvement in your girth. So, even with a solid abundance of fat genes, volition may determine a hefty trim look or a hefty obese slug appearance. It's your choice.

Fact Summary:

1. Genetically, we are all born with unequal potential in life.
2. Environmentally, we also begin life with unequal *opportunities.*
3. Although we're stuck with our inherited genes and initial environmental influences, volition—the will power of the mind—can greatly minimize the inequalities.
4. Your high fat potential at birth isn't a life sentence unless you don't *mind.*

CHAPTER 3

Medical Double-Speak

Thanks to medical science, physicians and nurse practitioners can keep us alive for twice as long as our grandparents lived just a few generations ago. We're healthier than ever, with immunizing vaccines that protect us from rapacious diseases that used to cruelly kill tens of thousands of our vulnerable ancestors. Medical advances in just the last century are beyond anyone's most fanciful expectation. To those early twentieth century physicians not that long ago, routine organ transplants, the Human Genome Projects, DNA accomplishments, computerized robotic surgery, powerful antibiotics, analgesics galore and even Dolly, the cloned sheep, were all science fiction. Medical science advancing into new-age bionic technology has made our lives infinitely healthier than we ever imagined. We can function virtually pain free, destroy most diseases with a trove of medications and there's boundless longevity.

Not so fast with your exuberance, folks. Medical technology is certainly praise-worthy. Unfortunately, consumers and too many practitioners aren't. Despite our miraculous brain and our ability to achieve technological Nirvana, we don't quite know how to use either.

There seems to be some sinister variable, some pitiable flaw in our human miracle that blocks a common sense, compassionate and more effective use of our incredible technology. Clearly, science can offer us unimagined health and fitness, and we can return the gifts with deep gratitude for all we have. We're more scientifically sophisticated than ever in the history of life. We know all about the foods that help and harm us. Our high school level First Aid courses teach us more about preserving and saving lives than the best of physicians knew a few generations ago. We know all about exercise as an integral ingredient to health and how sexually transmitted diseases can be easily prevented. We know about the use and abuse of medications and, of course, we're secure in our awareness that the medical profession has the capacity to effectively treat just about anything.

We know all this stuff, yet it has become kind of a *so what* since the vast majority of us, including the medical professionals, simply don't practice what is known. Worse yet, we tend to ignore what would unarguably enhance the health and fitness of ourselves and the rest of humanity. For those of you who don't already know all of this, here's a quick refresher and a chance for you to no longer ignore this stuff by taking it all for granted.

Since the discovery of the wonder drug, penicillin, in 1928, medical research's dogged persistence has blessed us with over a hundred additional kindred antibiotics capable of defeating just about every known bacterial infection and disease. In less than one hundred years, unstoppable infectious bacterial predators like pneumonia, tuberculosis, streptococcus and syphilis have surrendered to science's arsenal of antibiotics. We won the battles against infectious diseases.

At least we thought we did. But don't ever forget that taking our technology for granted is dangerous. It's recklessly haughty to assume we won the war just because we were victorious in some scientific battles. A little humility argues that the war against disease is postponed, but never won. That's because even victories can succumb to defeat without defensive vigilance.

Medical practitioners and consumers have been *abusing*, by inappropriately *using* antibiotics since penicillin imbued humanity with an everlasting gratitude that is waning with time by taking antibiotics for granted.

One of humanity's nasty streaks is greed, and another is naiveté. If one is good for you, two are better, and if it cures *this,* it's bound to cure *that*. Consequently, consumers have been gulping down these antibiotics like peanuts for all sorts of ailments even before they happened. Examples: On their way to brothels, servicemen have been popping penicillin to prevent VD for decades, while families have wonder pill orgies during flu season—even though antibiotics are useless against the flu viruses. And there are always physicians who will give you all the antibiotic prescriptions you want, just to shut you up, or because they don't know any better.

All of these abuses result in resilient bacteria developing mutant, resistant strains to survive antibiotic attacks. Humanity's gratitude is eroding, while deaths from infectious, bacterial diseases are again rising. It's a hit and hide guerrilla warfare that keeps assaulting medical knowledge and technology. We're beginning to lose many of those hard fought battles because too many of us have joined the enemy.

☙ ❧

Having explained all of the above, what do these revelations have to do with obesity? How about everything. Despite our awareness of obesity's friends and enemies, obesity is nearing epidemic percentages in the United States. We know eating too many calories and avoiding exercise are fattening. We know all about the food group pyramid, the dangers of trendy diets and *periodic* workouts. In other words with all our scientific information, we should know how to stay fit and healthy. The problem is that we store all worthwhile knowledge in the *take it for granted* section of our memory bank, and we get fat anyway. How come?

Here are some of the most obvious reasons, which are promoted by another tragic paradox. Each decade we are doing less and less, while eating more and more of the wrong foods, despite our sophistication to health hazards.

The contradiction becomes more understandable when medical doublespeak talks to us. We're told to stay healthy with exercise, moderate balanced meals and by resisting reliance on special diets and hunger-curbing drugs. On the other hand, for decades we have been pelted by a very different message, prompted by the pharmaceutical industry and eagerly endorsed by medicine. It goes something like this. You don't have to work hard to change or even feel better. There's a drug solution for just about every human problem or concern.

The pharmaceutical corporations court physicians with expensive meals, free samples and a variety of other incentives to order their products. The medical profession swoons at the courtship, and a drug dealer/pusher relationship is sealed.

Since the old Excedrin ads, drug marketing has become as common as beer commercials. If you're overweight, feel low, can't get it up, can't sleep or sleep too much, take a pill. There are plenty available and all you have to do is swallow. Take as directed and satisfaction is guaranteed, provided the side effects don't kill you. No need to redefine your lifestyle. Do it, whatever it is, the easy way.

Pills don't just discourage the effort and the pride in personal achievements; they have clearly contributed to street drug prosperity. Medicine pampers the demand side of the drug equation, both legal and illegal.

In addition to those unpredictable side effects, too often there's a much more pervasive downside. Taking a pill replaces a natural search for ways to more effectively cope with the stresses of everyday living. In discouraging problem solving behavior, the ease of popping a diet pill, for example, may further discourage exercise and permanent weight loss. There are infinitely more natural, enduring ways to lose weight than swallowing pills. And where's the personal satisfaction in temporarily reducing by pill, rather than positive changes in behavior.

଒ ଓ

Clearly there's both a legal and an illegal drug problem in the United States, and both *medicine* and the *pharmaceutical industry* remain principal conspirators in perpetuating the problem. Medicine's sincere opposition to illegal street drugs is unquestioned, even by me. The real issue, however, is medicine's double standard.

The cleverly devised and relentlessly executed marketing campaign to sell legal drugs for virtually every physical and emotional problem simultaneously sells an *idea.* It is an insidious paradox that drugs represent a magical shortcut to Nirvana. Such a doublespeak idea perpetuates the demand side of both legal and illegal drug abuse, and the war on drugs hopelessly flounders in a confusing web of friendly fire.

What a dilemma—you can get both indispensable, life saving drugs together with the feel-good or look-better pills from your friendly physician. Somehow the science of healing has gotten mixed up with the art of dealing, and everyone loses except, of course, the pharmaceutical suppliers.

☙ ❧

The *Physician's Desk Reference*, (PDR), provides legitimate-sounding words for diet pills. Under Obesity Management and Appetite Suppressants are such Methamphetamine related drugs as Desoxyn and Adipax-P. There are cautions all over the PDR about the addictive effects and other dangers from these drugs. Yet, all it takes to get them is an overweight, demanding patient and an easily intimidated or greedy, friendly physician. Ask Rush Limbaugh.

A recent article in *Time Magazine*, entitled "Fat Pill for Teens," may be providing another seemingly easy way out for chubby youth, especially those who love goodies and hate exercise. Xenical is an easy-to-take pill for a complex teenage problem. Sanjay Gupta, M.D., a CNN medical correspondent, acknowledges that the percentage of overweight teenagers has tripled since the 80's, with a corresponding increase in serious health problems like heart disease and diabetes. Originally marketed in 1999 for adults, the FDA approved Xenical in 2003 for adolescents. Dr. Gupta suggests that, as the first diet drug approved for youth, there's an outgrowth of current alarming obesity statistics in "our quick-fix society." He explains that, "the pill works by blocking an enzyme that absorbs fat," causing "gas, diarrhea and incontinence for kids who dip into fatty treats." The drug costs about $1,500 a year, and for adults, when Xenical use stopped, so did the weight loss. Maybe as a last resort for parents of genetically obese kids, diet pills are worth a try, but not as a substitute for exercise and sensible eating.

Then there are other more draconian medical treatments for obesity. These are the ones that really tend to turn my stomach. One medical procedure is called bariatric surgery, aka stomach bypass surgery, which is an impressive term for a desperate method of surgically reducing the size of one's stomach, generally with staples, partitions, etc…ugh. Even the president of the American Society for Bariatric Surgery, has a caution. Dr. Sugarman estimates that, out of the 110,000 gastric bypasses performed per year in the United States, one in five of the patients have complications. And for every 200 patients, "one to four" will die.

There's also the more popularized Liposuction for those hefties who finally decide all their accumulated fatty lumps have got to go the quick and expensive way. The fat is literally sucked out of your big, ah posterior, flaccid love handles or just about anywhere else the hidden fat is not so hidden.

Yet, as Dr. Samuel Klien, an obesity expert from Washington University in St. Louis, has discovered: vacuuming fat out of the obese has *solely* cosmetic value. He adds losing twenty pounds of fat by liposuction has no impact on metabolic health, including insulin resistance, inflammatory proteins, improved blood pressure, blood sugar, cholesterol or any other heart disease symptoms. Dr. Klein also confirms this book's repeated message that the magic formula for improving metabolic health is by simply eating less and exercising more.

An added irony is the fact that very few of us, or our kids, would need diet pills, invasive surgery, mockery or to endure early health problems if we had only learned to eat less and exercise more early in life. Daily habits are easiest to acquire or change when we're children. So parents beware, if your children are overweight, it's probably your fault.

Fact Summary:

1. Today's prudent application of medicine lags far behind the awesome advances in medical science and technology in the last hundred years.
2. Medicine is essential in treating your *matter*, while knowing little about your *mind*.
3. The medical and pharmaceutical institutions have a pusher/dealer relationship promoting a drug-dependent society.
4. Medicine preaches good health while offering too many drug solutions that interfere with healthy lifestyle changes.
5. Taking diet pills is no substitute for healthy exercise and sensible eating habits.
6. Einstein must have known about this chapter when he said, "Insanity is doing the same things over and over, while expecting a different result."

CHAPTER 4

Education's Misguided Priorities

This chapter was prepared especially for parents who believe our educational system knows what's best for the health and fitness of our kids. Throughout the history of our America, schools have been created to supplement the training and knowledge not offered by parents. In the very early years of our country, when wilderness areas were plowed into farmlands and proliferating homesteads coalesced into towns, learning farming and basic survival crafts from parents just wasn't enough. The growing social interdependency of humans meant sharing knowledge, skills and beliefs to ensure the prosperity of emerging communities.

Our pioneer ancestors were self-reliant in just about everything but harmonious community living. In towns, survival skills weren't quite as important as social skills that gradually redefined self-reliance. Adapting to and relying on others was becoming increasingly essential. Surviving in towns meant buying and selling goods or services, banking and sharing an endless fund of information from books. Social skills had become as necessary as survival skills, and most parents soon recognized that a basic prerequisite to community success was learning the *Three R's*. Education shifted from parents to churches to formal schools, where teaching reading, writing and arithmetic became as fundamental to urban survival then, as it is now. Since the birth of our nation the Three R's have remained as important as ever, however, teachers are missing a vital addition to our schools' Three R's.

Pioneers took very little for *granted*. Each day was a survival struggle, and each night they were grateful to be alive. Yet, in those early schools, teachers were aware that building communities demanded more than courage and stamina. Literacy was essential and the Three R's its key. Also, the last curriculum their students needed was a course in how to exercise. The long walks to and from school and their physically exhausting chores at home were no doubt enough of a workout. All of that has changed with modern urban priorities.

☙ ❧

How *not* to take our lives for *granted* is now vital to good health and fitness. And with today's convenience laden reliance on technology, exercise in school has become at least as essential as the Three R's.

When most of today's kids drive or are driven home from school, there are probably no chores, other than watching TV or fingering the computer while stuffing a few unneeded cookies down their gluttonous little throats. What a relaxing, indulgent life that relentlessly encourages kids toward a later life of fat and unhealthy.

Some of you may still cling to the argument that teaching kids the value of exercise by example is parents' responsibility, not the schools'. After all, parents are the supreme role model and master educators of their children—like it or not. This argument is absolutely true, while the readiness of most parents to teach or even encourage exercise is absolutely false.

Don't forget the original and most defensible purpose of schools is to teach what parents don't or can't.

In other words, without the Three R's in the school curricula, many kids would never learn how to read, write or balance the checkbooks they wouldn't have. The same goes for physical education. Without daily physical activity as part of a school's curricula, too many kids would grow fatter, flabbier and unhealthier because of fat, flabby, unhealthy parents disinterested in exercise.

Parents have an overpowering positive or negative relationship with their kids, which will be underscored in the next chapter. For now, accept the fact that parental influence is frequently detrimental to their children's health and welfare, while too many schools aren't much better in the roll of surrogate parents.

As Director of Physical Education at Skyline College in California, Bob Lualhati created a student fitness testing program over twenty years ago. His findings, based on the comprehensive measuring of 37,732 students, are a sobering eye-opener.

"Between 9/1/83 and 5/20/93," he begins, "our fitness testing data established that 8.9% of our population of Skyline students had Body Mass Index (BMI) of 30 or higher (morbidly obese). However, during the next ten years, the data points out that 14.2% of the Skyline students had BMI's of 30 or greater (almost doubling the percentage from the earlier decade). And the data for this semester (2005) is 16.9% of the students with BMI's of 30 or more."

Professor Lualhati's exhaustive research further reveals disturbing twenty-year trends for "over fat" and "obese" students. These findings are also of particular interest to parents and their kids.

Different from the more general BMI, these measurements of overfat and obese are more specifically defined by each person's "percent of fat content" or "Body Composition" (BC). A detailed explanation of the BC measurement is contained in Section K of the Appendix. Body Composition standards are also shown in Section L.

In Lualhati's research, using a twenty-year overweight (BMI) or overfat (BC) measurement, the outcomes are the same. The percentage of students at Skyline College who are overweight or overfat has increased dramatically since the original measurements in 1983. Based on cancer research, Lualhati adds that cancer potential increases 52% in males and 62% in females who are morbidly obese.

As a footnote, this data is from a college that constantly urges Physical Education. What about the schools that don't?

One part of a school program that is rarely neglected is *lunch*. That's when all the students hang out at the cafeteria buying what tastes good rather than what's good for them.

In past decades there have been some government and private health group efforts to pressure schools into healthier menus, especially in subsidized lunch programs for the poor. Such forays have had limited success, at least in part because students reject the nutritious stuff, and schools like to avoid student revolts. Then there are the many brown bag kids still into the baloney and mayonnaise sandwiches on white bread.

In recent years, organizations for healthful foods have rallied with even louder noise about nutritious lunch programs in schools and the elimination of those notorious soft drinks loaded with everything but good health. This counterattack on schools' resistance to healthful eating (and drinking) may be too little too late for our generation. It seems to be the seductive power of marketing over health, with marketing still ahead by a tray of greasy fries, burgers and a soft drink.

☙ ❧

The abundance of research documenting the increased obesity of American kids further highlights another problem. There are a substantial number of parents who aren't into preventive medicine. Throughout this book, the precious linchpin to good health and fitness is *preventing poor health.* That's what preventive medicine is all about. And if parents aren't concerned, why should their uninformed kids care? Here's a simple formula. More exercise + fewer calories = the most essential aspect of preventive medicine. Schools should post that formula in every classroom.

Along with inadequate physical education programs, it's painfully obvious that kids need to know symptoms of poor health and how to care for their bodies. If most parents aren't prepared to do it, we may need to teach kids to monitor their own health at an early age, like age five. The essential Three R's are of limited value if people don't know how to remain healthy. It's like learning a language is so much easier when you're an open and accessible five-year-old. I'm all for adding *preventive medicine* to the basic Three R's—the Three R's + PM.

By the time we reach adulthood and grasp the value of common sense, we can't figure out why more of us aren't into preventive medicine. That's simple—money-oriented marketing and technology has "seduced" us with quick-fix alternatives to common sense and good health—while too many of our "seduced" parents are poor role models. Those seductive marketing messages gradually wear down our resistance until we simply take for granted a life of "taste good" pleasure, comfort and convenience. Just as we have learned to thoroughly enjoy technological advances now taken for granted, marketing has further sweet-talked us into the cherished life of instant gratification.

So, our present version of common sense argues that feeling good for now is more important than preserving good health for later. Eating unhealthful, taste-great foods, or avoiding exercise to rest your overly rested body, clearly match the reasoning for *smoking* because it feels good or *condomless sex* because it feels better. We'll worry about lung cancer or AIDs later.

Sadly, it's hard to endorse common sense when feel good, quick fixes are convincingly peddled throughout modern urban society, from marketing moguls, to friends, peers and parents. We know it's bad for us but we do it anyway because it feels good now and everybody else does it—well, it seems like everybody else.

Come on, folks, that kind of common sense logic doesn't make any sense. Please pause here for a few moments and explore why you don't take better care of yourself and your family. In addition to the above bogus reasoning, you may expect science to find a cure for those ailments later or you might say it's your business and you choose to live for today, the hell with tomorrow. Such a philosophy is fine, provided you're clear about the consequences of bad habits and really don't mind "tomorrow" which, by the way, becomes today. And if you really believe you don't *mind*, you probably wouldn't be reading a book called *Minding Your Matter.*

Fact Summary:

1. Many parents don't teach nutrition or the value of exercise to their kids.
2. In schools, physical education is falling, while student obesity is alarmingly rising.
3. The term *preventive medicine* is vital to good health.
4. Since many parents don't practice preventive medicine, such a curriculum in schools is as important as the Three R's.
5. Too late for you? Not worth the effort? How about your kids?
6. Sooner or later, that "tomorrow" you're not worried about—is today!
7. Instant gratification is great—for an instant.
8. Obesity is no longer a middle age disease, as evidenced by the 1983 obesity mean age of 45 dropping to an average age of 28 in 2005!

CHAPTER 5

Make Sure Your Friends Really Are

Do you think you're smart? Compared to your ancestors you're probably brilliant. This is the Twenty-First Century overflowing with everything you've ever wanted to have or wanted to know. If there's something, anything, you don't have, turn on the "infomercials" and there's everything you'll never really need. If there's something you don't know, just hit the Internet and *voila*, you'll have the knowledge of a million libraries at your fingertips in minutes, rather than days, months or years.

There's just one problem that was noted in previous chapters. It's the enormous disparity between "knowing and doing." We know all about what's good for our health and fitness, yet that knowledge doesn't necessarily translate into doing anything about it.

This Twenty-First Century paradox of brilliantly knowing what's good for you while stupidly doing something else that isn't good for you, borders on some kind of craziness. Perhaps it's a loss of reality contact or some type of delusional thinking. Maybe it's a new form of Schizophrenia. More likely, it's some sort of culturally contagious behavioral problem.

Mental health professionals have a huge manual containing all the currently researched mental disorders. It's entitled *The Diagnostic and Statistical Manual of*

Mental Disorders (DSM). Currently it's the DSM IV, mentioned in an earlier chapter. Every few years researchers add a few more classifications. So, one of these days we'll have a DSM V.

Within the manual are all sorts of initials and acronyms for mental disorders. Along with ADHD (Attention Deficit Hyperactivity Disorder), PTSD (Post Traumatic Stress Disorder) and (GAD) Generalized Anxiety Disorder, we could add HAD, an acronym for Health Abuse Disorder. Such a disorder would fit over half of our population and enrich psychotherapy and the psychiatric pill business. It would also exonerate all of us with "it's not our fault, because it's a mental illness."

That kind of logic, however, is not very logical, since its basic premise is faulty word logic. HAD is not really a mental disorder and therefore doesn't warrant an excusable illness label. It's simply a mind problem that's pandemic in the modern urban world. HAD has become a fundamental part of our cultural development in a "feel good" society where indulging your mind and body with goodies overshadows eventual poor fitness or ill health. It is like the legends of Faust—pleasure now, pain later. No, we're not suggesting the stoic life of a monk. Just don't forget Aristotle and moderation, coupled with some independent common sense thinking.

Survival is no longer a major problem in our society. The problem today is relying too much on others at the expense of health and fitness. That's how we learn HAD and even the best of modern medicine can't keep us healthy when we remain willingly influenced by unhealthy lifestyles—and that's when we've been *had.*

"Aw, come on, one more beer ain't gonna hurt ya."

"There's another piece of chocolate pie left. No? Please don't disappoint me, honey. I know you can finish it."

"Don't worry about your diet. It'll keep until tomorrow. Have some more fettuccini; it's not that fattening."

"No, you're not getting fat. You look fine."

Sound familiar? It's not just professional marketing that influences what we do. We are constantly influenced by acquaintances, friends and family. Where do you think our biases, morality, habits, beliefs and food preferences come from? It doesn't matter if you agree. Just stay aware that if you tend to maintain eating and comfort behaviors contrary to good health, you're either self-indulgent, self-destructive or you just don't care.

Misery Loves Company was one of grandma's favorites, and it's still one of mine. Many drunks resent sober acquaintances, while most drunks trying to stay sober won't succeed as long as there are drinking friends around.

This premise also applies to fat people. Hang around gluttonous, couch potato friends who would rather drive than walk, and there's a high probability you'll end up a gluttonous, couch potato who'd rather drive than walk. That's, of course, unless you're one of those rare Alpha Dogs, capable of influencing others. Like it or not, there are leaders and followers in urban societies, and the huge majority of us are followers.

If you're one of the majority, make sure friends are positive role models with healthy lifestyles. Again, it's always your choice as long as you keep realizing that you actually have choices. If not, at least *choose* to avoid those "misery loves company" types.

☙ ❧

The toughest of all relationships to avoid are also the influences most difficult to resist. You simply weren't able to choose your family. Parents were the awesome, all pervasive authority during your most formative early years. Doesn't matter if it were a double or single parent family, if mom were an admired brain surgeon or a scorned junkie, there was no escaping her powerful influence. The same goes if dad were around or not around. Either way, you learned from both of them.

During those preadolescent vulnerable years of our lives, parents were always bigger, smarter, stronger and there—even when not there. Besides, we really needed them for most everything—for the survival basics of food, shelter, and protection—for emotional basics like expressions of love, caring and caressing, and for those attitudinal, moral and intellectual social skills. That's when parental disciplining and interacting branded each of us with a unique signature even if there was no direct guidance, no discipline and little interaction.

During that period of our lives, parents were the undisputed, most powerful and necessary authority in our narrow universe. We watched and listened even when we didn't know we were watching and listening. What our parents did or didn't do etched an everlasting impression on our developing psyches. Our empty little computers were hungrily downloading significant aspects of our environment, and parents were the most significant, the most indispensable of all aspects.

OK, that's enough. You get the point. All of your parents' habits, attitudes, interests and activities profoundly influenced you, and even today there's no escape from those early learnings, including eating and exercise habits.

I still feel irrationally uneasy unless I finish everything on my plate. Dear old mom hammered that command into my memory bank over seventy years ago. In lieu of psychotherapy, a fair solution for me has been to begin with smaller plates of food.

We're all faced with the same immutable quandary. How do we overcome those inevitably negative parental influences that seem glued to our brain? That's a good question, but what about the parents who are a positive health influence? Well, those kids are the fortunate ones—provided their parents aren't serial killers or flawed in other ways.

We're simply not born into urban society with equal genetics or parents, and our defensive strategy in dealing with those variable influences is the focus of what's left of this chapter.

Trading your health indifferent parents in on better ones was not an option, at least during those early, formative years of your life. That's when you began to wonder why your family was so soft and round—when other kids may have made fun of you, which was puzzling at first, then frustrating later as you sought refuge with other soft round kids. By the time you reached your teen years, you tended to huff and puff your way through life's routines, as you unwittingly mirrored your parents' soft and round lifestyles.

Remember, you can't *not* be influenced by your parents' behaviors. You can, however, openly resist with a counter phobic, reverse influence strategy. If you used that approach you may have become one of the angular and firm. Being healthy and fit because your parents led unhealthy, round and soft lifestyles does occur, albeit occasionally. That's one of those exceptions to the rule.

But cheer up, folks. Regardless of your girth and flab index, you're not trapped. Being overweight and under-exercised is not a life sentence.

One of the miraculous aspects of your body is its fluid obedience to its leader, meaning you, not your parents. Admittedly, it's a lot easier to change when you're six rather than sixty, especially if your family and thin genomes are rooting for you. Still, if you're able to think for yourself, there's always room for change in the condition of your body's health and fitness. You just have to know how.

Here are a couple of contrasting scenarios to clarify the essence of positive behavioral change.

Subject A had been living under the influence of fat genes, obese parents and their sluggish lifestyle throughout his entire twenty years. Unthinkingly, he adapted predictably well to genetic and parental influences. It's a no-brainer. Such a person keeps doing what he's doing or not doing with no expectation of any change. For Subject A, change is no longer even a tiny radar blip of possibility. He/she has absently accepted fat and its lifestyle.

For the first twenty years of his life, Subject B's scenario was ostensibly the same—the relentless influence of fat genes, fat parents and resultant unhealthy lifestyles. The outcome, however, was markedly different. At age twenty-one, Subject B decided he really disliked huffing and puffing his way through life with a round and soft mirror image. Dissatisfaction with his fitness was the catalyst egging him on to try something else. Gradually he altered his lifestyle, his huffing and puffing disappeared and his distasteful mirror image morphed into something quite tolerable. No, he'll never be an Olympic athlete or svelte male model. He just looks and feels better, firmer, more self confident and certainly healthier!

What's the difference in these two scenarios? None, as long as we solely focus on the body's helpless conformity to fat genes and bad habits. Once we take a good look at ourselves and dislike what we see, the operative terms for change are personal responsibility, thinking and expectations—mind over matter!

Subject A adapted without consciously thinking about choices—kind of a fatalistic view with no change expectations and no personal responsibility. He just was what he was and there was nothing he could do about it, even if he wanted to, which never really occurred to him.

Subject B also adapted well to fat for twenty years, until it dawned on him that the mind is in charge of his body, his mind and no one else's.

Your body is a genuine follower, awaiting orders from your mind. Yet your mind is also somewhat of a follower in being influenced by what others do and say.

What I'm getting at is this. The input of opinions and biases from friends, teachers and parents will shape your own opinions, biases and expectations. These influences aren't truths; they are simply opinions and biases that may sadly narrow your expectations of your own potential. Each of us, as individuals, has no choice but to recognize the influence of others. Then ask yourself what you need to survive most efficiently. This will help identify friends from foe. As long as you assume full responsibility for your own health and fitness, sorting out good from bad influences will be much easier.

Once again, your mind controls your body, so take that responsibility seriously or other minds will do it for you.

Fact Summary:

1. HAD or health abuse disorder means doing what's bad for your health despite knowing how to make it better.
2. Some friends, as well as marketers, clearly contribute to your HAD.
3. Parents are the most powerful influence over your matter, mind and the presence or absence of HAD.
4. Disliking how you feel and what you see in the mirror are the essential steps toward assuming personal responsibility for your health and fitness.
5. In controlling your health, your mind is more powerful than your parents. So, use it!

Part II

Know Yourself and How You Affect Your Health and Fitness

Chapter 6

What are You?

What a way to start a new chapter, with a trick question. Modern day experts can offer us sophisticated, scholarly theories about who or what we really are, while the grim truth is, we don't know. Maybe taking ourselves for granted has protected us from caring, or maybe Popeye had the right answer all along. "I yam what I yam."

Randomly ask the average adult what they really are, and invariably the initial reply is wide-eyed astonishment, followed by a wide-eyed question—something like, "What do you mean?"

When you repeat the question with no further clues, a variety of stereotypical answers follow:

"Aaah. I'm an American."

"Well, we're all human beings."

"I'm an educated woman."

"You mean like my religion? I'm a Christian."

"I don't know; what are you?"

The average person won't mention the word *miracle*, and there won't be any display of goose pimpled "awes" or "awesomes" in their replies. We're just too used to ourselves to notice.

It's like trying to define health. Clearly, good health is cherished by all, yet no one truly appreciates good health until they're sick or disabled. Since we're all very good at defining pain and discomfort, the absence of bad health is no doubt our best definition of good health. We simply don't consciously feel good about our good health; we just have it. We take it for granted, as we do ourselves, until we're on the brink of losing it. Then, like Gollum's ring, we want it back.

All of this underscores the purpose of Part II, which is to help us preserve or reclaim our health by getting to know the value of what we may lose. It begins by knowing what we are. Most of us know others much better than we know ourselves. That makes us vulnerable and summons another grandma-ism: "You can be your own best friend or your worst enemy."

ꙮ ꙮ

As you might have guessed from the title of this book, we are mind and matter, with our health relentlessly monitored by the mind. But don't take my word for it.

Again, at the risk of lecturing you into a deep sleep, brace yourself while I toss a little science and research your way. Bear with me for a page or two.

Much of what this book is about is contained in one of the dictionary's longest words, *Psychoneuro-immunology*. It's a relatively new science that investigates our four interacting information-processing systems. They include the mind, the endocrine system, the nervous system and the immune system. These four interactive systems are in constant collaboration with each other. What matters (pardon the pun) for this book is how the first system, the *mind*, influences the other three systems, our *matter*.

Current scientific research agrees that the brain system is the physiological correlate of the mind, and the first line of defense against an ill, aging or dying body. As important, it's the body's principle health and well being advocate—or enemy.

Scientists from virtually all disciplines now recognize that our beliefs influence the biology of our body. The electrical and chemical activity in the brain's nerve cells represent our changing beliefs and thoughts. This is the process that is also changing our biology. In responding to the brain, however, the body can't interpret the nature of the psychological activity. The body doesn't know if the belief is fact or fiction, good or bad. Simply put, the body responds helpfully or harmfully to the electrical brain activity, not the psychological thought. The polygraph (lie detector) is a good example. It doesn't detect lies; it displays neurochemical, circulatory and respiratory responses to thoughts. Then the real art, not science, is trying to figure out if the readout squiggles represent lies.

In science, these findings—that our beliefs influence our biology—are considered *biopsychosocial* if any reader is still awake enough to care.

There's an abundance of scientific research verifying how mind thoughts are converted into lasting body changes. An example is four indispensable coping skills that can consciously control the condition of our bodies. These are knowledge (about our world), inner resources (beliefs, biases, etc.), social support (relationships with friends, groups, loved ones) and spirituality (religious beliefs, etc). All four coping skills are clearly linked to such bodily outcomes as resistance to physical illness, improved immune system function and increased longevity, provided such coping efforts are *positive*.

Enough of these research details. So, back to small words and huge ideas. Slashing through the dense underbrush of scientific papers loaded with big charts, big numbers and bigger words, the message is clear and simple. You are capable of being your own best friend or worst enemy. Get to know yourself. Start with the miracle of your mind and body and the perils of taking either for granted. Do that much and regardless of how you're defined, you may begin to realize that only you are responsible for your health and fitness.

There are cultural implications to what we are, which has a lot to do with where we are. Culture sprinkles all kinds of adjectives into the identity equation. Short, tall, fat, skinny, pretty, ugly, handsome, frumpy, funny, boring, sexy, etc., etc., etc. If you pride yourself with a good sense of humor in the United States, don't be too surprised when you can't find a laugh or even a grin in other cultures. Observe those hilarious comedians in Cuba, Austria or Swaziland and your reactions will range from unfunny, to strange, to childish, to downright disgusting.

We are big on appearance in this country. Thin is definitely in—while stout is out.

In parts of Asia and elsewhere in our small world, thin fashion models are a revolting turnoff. Fat is eye-popping sexy in Afghanistan. The bones through the nose and plates through the ear lobes aren't our brand of beauty either, even though there is a subculture of ours hanging things through all sorts of body parts.

The human genome doesn't seem to have a universal beauty gene. What we do have is thirty thousand genes that we know very little about, yet how we process information assures us there must be genes for adaptation and learning. History also keeps showing us that much of our self-image is shaped by the culture in which we live and learn.

What we learn also includes what we eat which will be thoroughly served in the next chapter.

Fact Summary:

1. The condition of your body clearly echoes your state of mind.
2. A major obstacle to preserving good health is taking it for granted.
3. Worldly knowledge, beliefs, relationships and spirituality profoundly affect your biology.
4. Our culture has a powerful influence over our mind and body.
5. With countless adjectives describing what you are, just remember you are what you believe you are. You're a miracle, so think positive.

CHAPTER 7

You Are What You Eat

"Hey, Mom, what's for dinner?"

"One of your favorites, Honey. We're having roast leg of dog. It's from a tender little terrier."

"What else?"

"Well, we've got plenty of noodles, bamboo shoots, pickled snake and deep fried grasshoppers; and for dessert, we'll have glazed grubs."

"Oh boy, thanks, Mom."

Sound tasty? Not likely, unless we're from parts of Asia or Africa. Yet, no matter where in the world we're born, we all have nearly the identical anatomy and physiology. So why do some of us salivate with delight while others wretch with disgust at the sheer thought of such a nourishing, protein rich meal? The answer underscores the supreme power of the human mind. It's not the meal we're judging. It's the thought of the meal. It's our mind performing one of its many functions. In fact, our mind blends so inseparably with our body, a brief review of how the mind works will provide an important gateway into the secrets of controlling our health and fitness.

A thought is a fundamental part of our mind. It is an infinite and amorphous reservoir of all we learn and all we come to know in our lives. This mind of ours begins with nothing more than the miraculous ability to organize and process information received from our sensations and perceptions, which are some of those other components of the mind.

More to the pragmatic point, the mind allows us to learn everything from verbal symbols such as language, to what's right and wrong, good and bad, ugly and pretty, tasty and nasty, fun and drudgery, stressful and tranquil. By the time the human mind, this miracle of all miracles, reaches puberty, it's teeming with a special language: identity, biases, prejudices and every other mental activity that makes us so special.

How we register, store and retrieve all this information is another mind-boggling function called *memory*. Without it, humans would be unable to profit from the past or anticipate the future. There'd be no meaningful understanding of life's perpetual situations. We simply wouldn't learn from our experiences. We would be reduced to biological impulses and instincts. And that's far less than human.

We are also the only species able to *adapt* to any environment, despite our puny strength, unremarkable agility and thin, fragile skin. In the animal kingdom, the most physically *powerful* predators of the world haven't a chance against humans who are the most *adaptable* predators in the world. Unfortunately, adaptability can also be our enemy when we adapt to bad habits. Once we have innocently and unwittingly succumbed to a "bad habit" we tend to perpetuate what's not good for us by enlisting another extraordinary ability of the mind. It's called *rationalization,* one of our overused defense mechanisms.

Humans have an uncanny ability to create all kinds of plausible reasons for sustaining harmful habits, especially eating habits, the target of this chapter. When we rationalize that the bad habit is really okay, or beyond our control, rationalization becomes our enemy.

Because of our mind's indispensable power to control everything we do, the mind must be an indelible part of every chapter in this book. Its awesome power can be used either for our health as friend, or against us as enemy. Everyone with a normal mind has the responsibility to care for themselves, and how we use our mind to regulate what we eat, clearly represents how well we are caring for ourselves. It's always our choice.

☙ ❧

To further explain similarities and differences in cultural eating habits, we need to start at the cave-dwelling beginning. How did we choose our food before society began choosing it for us? Well, put yourself in the place of your ancestors of a few million years ago. Not too different from us, they probably learned from their parents, who were busily avoiding being a flesh-eating dinosaur's entree. Otherwise, the only choices in those days were to eat whatever was available in their immediate surroundings, including flesh-eating dinosaurs if they got lucky.

Then, how did these primitive cave dwellers survive beyond their breast fed infancy? Their food availability and choices were no doubt extremely limited. Yet, even then there were choices that provided all they needed to sustain life, which prompts another critical question. Our hunch is that initial trial and error undoubtedly played an indispensable role in defining their eating habits. So, how did they know what to eat to keep them alive and reasonably well? If they tried a little of Plant X and they died or got sick, Plant X is off their menu.

Arguably, our cave-dwelling ancestors were omnivorous by necessity. They were prepared to eat plants, as well as animals, and as important, they were probably able to biologically sense what their bodies needed to compensate for nutritional deficiencies. Since they were still exclusively into *need* rather than *want*, they could selectively regulate health needs by eating some sort of vitamin-rich root, along with protein-rich flesh.

So, how come we salivate to the thought of eating a cute little lamb and gag if cute little dog is on the same menu? There's a long, convoluted physiological, psychological and theological answer that might put you to sleep. The short-term version is more than sufficient. In urban society, our eating habits, as well as our fashions, are parented by marketing and tradition with the distinction between need and want long out of focus.

Our eating habits and preferences remain a combination of learning and availability of edibles. At the same time, we're so caught up in what we've learned to eat, we have just about lost our ability to biologically know what foods we *need* to stay healthy. If, for some remote reason, you disagree, try some leg of dog or some delicious candied grubs.

☙ ❧

You sophisticated seniors and concerned parents of vulnerable overweight kids please pay attention. Since both groups have plenty to learn or unlearn about urban living, this is one of the most important lessons in this book crammed with important lessons. In fact, it's important enough to repeat occasionally. *The most insidious and persuasive enemy to our health and fitness is the ubiquitous marketing industry, virtually compelling you to buy what you don't need, to worship comfort and to restrict your freedom of choice.* Just in case you've already forgotten, put this in your memory bank. If you don't *mind your matter*, others will be happy to mind it for you.

Humans are super quick studies. We learn fast, which is a genuine plus. We are also highly suggestible, which can be a genuine minus. Tell us over and over again that something will make us feel better, more comfortable, happier, prettier. When that happens it's just a matter of time before we're hooked and we've really learned to need the stuff. There are no exemptions, no one's immune. It's like a weapon of mass destruction, only more subtle, sinister, disarming. Marketing is a pervasive mist that chokes off the freedom of choice as it settles over us so-called sophisticated humans. It's a science of influence and persuasion. That would be just fine, except too frequently the influence favors an unhealthy way of living.

Marketing strategies were never developed to tell the truth, they were always designed to sell a product. Marketers have become so good at what they do, they qualify as world-class illusionists. They deal in deception, exaggeration, promises, distortions, half-truths and downright lies. Marketing everything from tiny widgets we don't need to gas-guzzling SUV's we really, really don't need, is the foundation of our nation's economic growth.

Marketers are legitimate business folks who are pretty much the same as their historical prototypes. Those were the *snake oil drummers* peddling a wide variety of alcoholic-laced *elixirs.* Those bottled potions were guaranteed to heal everything from the gout to syphilis. Whether they were labeled drummers, hucksters, peddlers, marketers or the more euphemistic sales representatives, they all wanted you to buy something and they didn't particularly care if you needed it or not. The business hasn't changed. It's just so much more clever, convincing and *sophisticated.*

ℭ ℵ

Since all urban dwellers eat, one of the most profitable products in urban society is food. The basic need to eat has not too surprisingly become a zillion dollar supply side marketing industry. Of course, simply supplying the consumers' need for food was never enough for marketers. The real profit is in manipulating the demand side by creating a compulsive desire for special foods. Thanks to marketing, we have not only been told what foods are supposed to be good for us, even if they're not, we've been taught to eat more than we need and to value taste over nutrition.

For most of us modern humans immersed in First World plenty, the constant struggle for survival long ago retreated into someone else's history. We're now free to eat anytime we choose, and we're encouraged to eat all the time. We can also eat just about anything we want, while programmed to eat only certain things. Roast leg of dog isn't on our psychological menu, but there are plenty of fried hamburgers dripping with saturated fats, Low Density Lipoproteins (LDL's), good old sodium and an abundance of calories.

There are several major reasons why hamburgers are so tempting. They're cleverly and relentlessly marketed until a hamburger with French fries represents the all American meal, anytime, day or night. It's replacing our traditional patriotic apple pie. Now it's good ole mom, the American flag and hamburgers. And all that salt and fried fat taste sooo good.

McDonald's, Jack in the Box, Wendy's, Burger King and Dairy Queen, to mention a few, have been feeding you seductive messages long before you downed your first greasy fix. The supply and demand concept presented in Economics 101 removed free choice from the equation long ago. If there's no demand, the suppliers will create one, and like a symbiotic marriage, they will take good care of each other. While the supply side gets richer, the demand side gets fatter.

You may be old enough to remember McDonald's big celebration back in the 70's, when, after a few years in business, they sold their millionth hamburger. Well, compared to now, that's hardly a blip of saturated fat on an MRI screen. If there were Nobel prizes for marketing, McDonald's would be a prime candidate. They are presently selling 600 million Big Macs to United States users each year! That doesn't include the other Macs, the cheaper ones, the double-patty ones, all sharing a common bond of tasty saturated fats and plenty of salt. Don't cringe in amazement yet. That statistic was just the tip of an unhealthy, overly salted iceberg. Add all those other fast food burger-pushers and the number of hamburgers downed by us Americans rockets well into the stratosphere. Then add the twenty billion hot dogs we consume yearly and you can start shaking your head off in amazement.

As you may have guessed, McDonald's didn't stop their burger pitch at our borders. Foreign nations throughout the world are gobbling up McDonald's marketing genius and Big Macs. In 2003, McDonald's was serving an incredible forty-six million customers a day at thirty thousand restaurants in one hundred nineteen countries. That's another head shaker.

Hooking kids on burgers is a lot easier than turning them onto cigarettes or street drugs. Burgers are legal for youth of any age, and kids are lured by pervasive advertising long before they can read. Addicted parents also represent the most convincing pushers. Soothing your screaming kid while downing your own burger and fries is a cinch. Just stuff a piece of fry or burger meat in baby's gaping mouth and the little tike will quickly learn from nurturing parents that salt, red meat and grease are yummy. Then, in a year or two, the little tot will be ordering his very own.

When I was one of those tots, years and years ago, marketing and habits created some powerful associations that linger on today—pork chops and applesauce, turkey and cranberry sauce, Valentine's Day and candy, Mothers' Day and Hallmark cards, Halloween and pumpkins and the more sinister associations like coffee and cigarettes or burgers, fries and cola. That might be why older kids, about to make their "own" food decisions, go for the burger and fries with a cola (rather than milk). Incidentally, an eight-ounce glass of cola has 100 calories, 27 grams of sugar and no calcium. In addition to being an unhealthy drink, it's outrageously expensive, since it costs a penny or so to make.

☙ ❧

It's not just the craze for fast food hamburgers invading our eating habits. Pizza marketing has gained an enviable foothold in the United States, where we munch down more Italian pizzas in a week than Italy probably gobbles up in a year.

"Hey, let's get a pizza!" is another unhealthy alternative to cooking dinner. Any leftovers, you can eat in the morning for breakfast. It's another WMD, well disguised to easily bequile the greedy undisciplined. There's nothing sneaky about the meal. It's right out there in the open, with marketing the major delivery system. Its message of mass destruction appeals to a special audience more interested in convenience and taste than health. Marketers do extremely well, because they're motivated by an old, well-quoted premise that, *There's a sucker born every minute.* The implication is that greedy, suggestible people wanting something for nothing are easy marks by hustlers with the alluring pitch they can give a lot of something for practically nothing. If it sounds too good to be true, it probably is. Related to eating, there's another caveat. If it tastes too good to be healthy, it probably isn't.

That's unless you're an Aristotle fan. Well over two thousand years ago this exceptionally wise philosopher prescribed a life of moderation. This is advice today's physicians should give all their patients. Unfortunately, moderation requires some regulation of our behavior that requires some personal responsibility—probably a real obstacle to our special audience. A monthly, or even bimonthly, pizza fix won't hurt you, but if marketing had its way, you would have pizza daily.

Before some reader insists that all pizzas aren't bad for you—I, and the entire scientific community, agree. Of course, all products ushered into your mouth aren't comparably harmful to your health. Assuming we are all equally vulnerable to the same stuff entering our mouth, filtered cigarettes are less damaging than the same unfiltered tobacco. Beer is less harmful than the same amount of bourbon, and certainly one cigarette or one bottle of beer a day is much less harmful to the body than a pack of cigarettes or seven beers.

Such common sense applies to food as well. The more pizza you eat, the less healthy it is for you, yet a veggie pizza with mushrooms, onions, artichokes and bell peppers sure beats one with pepperoni, ham, sausage and "extra cheese, please."

Incidentally, the one thing burgers and pizza have in common is one of our most "taken for granted," indispensable foods. It's called flour. Think burger, pizza, peanut butter and jelly or bologna, and they're all typically surrounded by flour, as bread, buns or crust. However, even those commercial forms of flour run the full range of nutritional value—from virtually nothing to something. Whole grain wheat flour is markedly more nutritious with fewer calories, than highly refined white flour. It's also noted that most pizzas are crusted with white flour.

Just don't let color alone fool you. Many whole wheat looking commercial breads are made with caramelized (dyed) white flour. Just keep reading those nutritional facts on the wrappers.

Resisting life's endless temptations requires at least a tad of personal responsibility, a dash of self-discipline and a liberal use of common sense. However, for many of those *suckers born every minute*, such mental coping behaviors may require too much effort and not enough pay-off. For them, it's not worth giving up a life of excessive comforts, a nice, easy, slow pace and fast foods. They've adapted to that passive way of living, and for now, it feels good. Flab, obesity and clogged arteries may take awhile to show them something is very wrong. By then, thanks to marketing, correcting a poor lifestyle that leads inextricably to poor health may be too difficult or too late.

There must be some meal immune to the magic of marketing moguls who sacrifice your homeostasis for a bigger profit margin. It's breakfast, of course—that important first meal of the day. It's the meal that prepares your entire body with vital nutrients that constitute the day's fuel. It's the food to get you started and keep you going, the wake-up meal to preserve your health and ignite your energy. It's just got to be the most nutritious of all meals.

In Twenty-First Century America, bacon and eggs are out and cereals are in. Cereals are the chosen breakfast for about fifty per cent of our nation. Unfortunately, that essential first meal can be a bowl of unnourishing, yet healthful expectations. Shame on us for our gullibility, and for parents' abusive permission to let their kids choose their cereals.

The frustrating truth is, breakfast is no more of a marketing free zone than any other meal. Cereal is a multibillion-dollar industry, luring consumers by colorful and cutesy packaging, palatable taste and a sprinkle of token nutrition. Marketing is more concerned that you're hooked than healthy, and cereal conglomerates are keenly aware that nutrition isn't particularly tasty.

The major addictive ingredients in cereals happen to be sugar and salt. But, you argue, refined sugar provides needed energy; while salt is a necessary blood pressure regulator and water balancing mineral. That's fairly accurate as far as it goes, which isn't far enough. The toxic effects of sugar and salt are also well documented and infinitely more disturbing.

Running down the medical alphabet, it becomes distastefully apparent that regularly downing excessive amounts of sugar can promote everything from acne outbreaks to yeast infections. Even more sinister, refined sugar, in particular, contributes to a weird yo-yoing of blood sugar chemical levels and an involuntary "need to eat" signal. Frequently, the result is an all too common condition in the United States called "binge eating." Even the American Medical Association recognizes that sugar can easily become a metabolism disrupter. The AMA goes as far as recommending a careful monitoring of one's sugar and concentrated starch intake.

Salt is equally necessary and dangerous to your health and girth. Asthma, congestive heart failure, hypertension and kidney problems are a few of the ailments promoted or aggravated by table salt. Again, the most harmful aspect of these two chemicals isn't their inherent toxicity; it's their addictive properties. Like alcoholics, many of us develop such a craving for sugar or salt, nothing seems to taste right without them, plenty of them.

In cereals, much of the stuff that enhances good health has been refined out, while sugar and salt are processed in. Of course, some cereals are more beneficial than others; and thanks to parents and marketing strategies, less popular—especially with kids. Shredded wheat has no saturated fat, no sodium, no sugar and no popularity. How many people do you know eat shredded wheat? I don't know any. However, I'll most likely get to know some in the future, since there's a new *frosted* shredded wheat on the market, and you know what *frosted* means.

Then there's Coco Pebbles with a gram of fat, one hundred eighty milligrams of sodium and twelve grams of sugar, yummy! CoCo Roos are even yummier with one hundred ninety milligrams of salt and fourteen grams of sugar. The list of desserts, disguised as cereals, seems endless. Drop into any supermarket and scan the cereal section. You'll find Cocoa Dyna-Bites, Reese's Puffs, Chocolate Mud and Bugs, Honey B's, and Oreo O's, to mention a few. Poor kids, how can they resist, especially when mom implies it's okay to get hooked. Worry about your health and excess weight later.

Granted, there are worse foods in your supermarket that will hook you faster and damage your health sooner. Yes, there's always something in urbania that's worse than something else, which isn't the point here. Breakfast cereal is hyped as the most nourishing food to start the day. As little tots all over the nation climb up their chairs to pound on the table with their big spoons, they're learning a grim, lip-smacking lesson—Mom's right, so believe what you hear from marketers.

I doubt that any tots are reading this book. I sure hope their parents are. You folks are the ones who can guide your children into a lifestyle of self-regulating fitness and good health, or one of chronic habituation to the lure of marketing distortions. That's not a healthy path for you or them.

Fact Summary

1. You weren't born with beliefs or food addictions. You learn them from parents, friends and marketers, whose own food biases can be harmful to your health and fitness.
2. Marketers aren't necessarily concerned with your health or fitness.
3. Many serious medical conditions are triggered or exacerbated by what you've learned to eat. The responsibility to eat right is yours, no one else's.

4. Food marketers promote taste, not nutrition, which usually means too much salt, sugar and fat. Deciding which foods are best for you is, again, your responsibility.
5. The only issue that's not your responsibility is trusting others to assume responsibility for you.
6. Taking for granted all one knows about health and nutrition is a serious health hazard.
7. The National Academy of Sciences, Institute of Medicine concluded in 2004 that the media, especially TV, affects children's (food) choices and may have a strong influence on their tendency toward obesity and chronic disease. Summarized, they were telling kiddy food marketers—back off!
8. A year later, the corporate cereal marketers launched an advertising campaign praising the health ingredients in "Cocoa Puffs," "Cinnamon Toast Crunch" and "Count Chocula." Their paraphrased reply to the National Academy of Sciences—says who?

CHAPTER 8

You Are What You Do

…and what you *do* can make an incredible difference in how you feel about what you *are*.

Defining what you actually are by what you do is the clearest, most defensible assessment of any individual. No psychologist, psychoanalyst, psychiatrist or even a good bartender could hope to devise a more accurate and reliable method of evaluation.

What you do means the way you behave regularly. Those high probability behaviors define what you are. They are the behaviors that keep cropping up even when you're unaware of them. Monitor and record your regular behaviors carefully and you'll come up with a psychological fingerprint, a behavioral DNA. They will also tend to confirm or refute all those nice things you say about yourself.

It's pretty foolproof. "I don't really drink that much," is easily verified by what you typically do. Get drunk several days a week and you're a drunk. Go to several movies a week and you're a movie buff, even if you keep telling everyone you much prefer reading. Sit at home most of the time watching TV and you're a couch potato, and if you constantly interrupt others when they're trying to tell you something, you're no doubt some kind of a jerk.

We can so easily deceive others and ourselves by what we say, while the charade ends with the doing. A dear, trusted friend of mine once adamantly insisted she never snored, until I tape-recorded the sounds. End of denials.

Grandma was right. "Don't tell me, show me," she used to say. She was a tough one to con. As suggested earlier, however, we bright humans are also highly suggestible or just plain gullible. We tend to listen to the words but not the behavioral music. We believe the spoken word for two principle reasons. When what we're told seems to be to our advantage, or the words are so convincing we overlook the music, we want to believe those genuine behaviors. Good ole marketers, they tell us what we want to hear in a super convincing way. That's why we all need to be more like grandma.

So, beginning at the root of the problem, check your behavioral DNA. It may pry some of your self-defeating illusions loose!

Here's a game for you if you're interested in what you really are. It's called Twenty Values. It's a game we used to play with Peace Corps trainees to help them see if their most typical behaviors were compatible with their assignment as a volunteer in a certain foreign country. Example, if a trainee's most valued everyday behaviors were focused on water sports like swimming, surfing, etc., an inland assignment in the Botswana Kalahari Desert might be a problem.

Try it with family and friends. Simply list the twenty activities you value most in your life. The ones you truly enjoy doing or just compulsively keep doing because the activity is regularly on your mind. Then list the top five, place a dollar sign in front of any that cost money to engage in the activity, "P" for any requiring other people, and an "S" for solitary. In a later chapter, the game's diagnostic usefulness will be critiqued. For now, suffice it to say, the game's therapeutic value sure beats Monopoly.

☙ ❧

Keeping in mind that you are what you regularly do, anyone who negatively influences what you do, represents an enemy to your health and welfare. That nice neighbor down the street that gives you a free hit of methamphetamines to help you feel better, may gradually hook you on an expensive addiction and deteriorating behavior. Street drug pushers are the more obvious, in your face enemies to healthy behavior.

Then there are the legitimate marketers who enthusiastically sell you an endless variety of legal, socially acceptable items that may subtly lead to unhealthy ways of living. Like it or not, these marketers may be one of your worst enemies, because the stuff they sell is so neat, so legal and effective in altering many of your most healthful activities. You are what you do; yet your behavior is powerfully influenced by what others say.

So, what are some of the ways modern day marketers have surreptitiously changed what we do? The real irony is that the most serious and insidious marketing changes in what we do can easily be described as what we don't do.

Let's refer back to the Prologue for a brief review. Remember that cherished miracle, ourselves? We are an inexplicably complex, astonishingly well-organized human life form, a neurobiochemical miracle that can do just about anything except understand itself. A casual look beneath our skin covering reveals a remarkable network of muscles, tendons and ligaments capable of withstanding the force of fierce, destructive hurricanes or sewing the most delicate patterns of thread into intricate mosaics of incredible beauty.

Understanding how and why we were created in the first place may have infinitely more to do with faith than science, yet from the size and strength of our heart and lungs to the power of our muscles, there's purpose. Nothing random or accidental here. We were designed as a thinking, procreating, compassionate miracle, with the ability to move around, representing one of our most essential behaviors. Take a quick gander at any anatomy book and you'll find that the most massive internal molecules are blood vessels to keep us functioning and muscles to keep us moving.

Now do a cursory comparison of your activity rates and those of your parents and grandparents. You will no doubt find that we are slugs compared to them. We are what we do, and we don't do much anymore. Humans were designed to move, and our ancestors rarely stopped. The kids played games like hopscotch, one foot off the gutter, hide and seek, as well as the major sports. These weren't compulsory school activities; they were popular after school events. Those were the days when you could hear mothers all over the neighborhood calling their kids to dinner.

For adults, one of their most typical activities in those days was walking and such variations as dancing, swimming, ice skating, bowling, roller skating and riding bicycles with one-to-one gears. Those were family activities. Just about every age was a participant, and no one minded the six or seven block walk to the movies.

Today when we leave the house, walking is not a viable option. We may run out of gas searching for the nearest parking place. Walking a few blocks is out of the question. There are more vehicles than people in most cities, and even church goers have disavowed the value of walking a few blocks to church. Sadly, through the power of the masses, it has become legal to double park in front of your church despite traffic jams. Parking in the center of the street is another common city alternative to public transportation or parking several blocks from church.

What happened in just a couple of generations to drastically change our mobility behaviors, to alter the use of our musculature? Technology happened, too quickly. Too much technology. Too much marketing of technology. When the present generation leaves the house, walking is no longer a natural travel option. The car is—our car does the walking for us. Marketing has encouraged us to get in a car and stay there.

Here's another statistical fact. Today, America has more registered cars than people licensed to drive them! Translated, this means there are more vehicles than drivers in most cities.

Why walk when you can drive?

Marketing has encouraged us to trade in walking for driving. Get in your car, get there quicker and preserve your energy is the subliminal message. Speed, convenience and comfort are the seductive and contradictory marketing mantras, selling everything from computers to SUVs. Get to where you're going fast, so you can kick back and rest your body when you arrive. Once home, only the most minimal movements are necessary. The fast food and frozen food markets permit meal preparation in minutes, thanks to micro-waves. Big affordable TV's have generously contributed to our greatly reduced outside activities. Thanks to cable and satellite TV, those past ventures outside to the movies are now more typically ventures to the living room. An added incentive to living room viewing is the cost of eating popcorn at home. It's a lot cheaper and you barely have to move to "nuke" it.

Tired of TV? Computers are an alternative in-house activity to keep you safely at home where you can conserve those muscles you rarely use. Perhaps you've also noticed that none of these technological advances require standing. In fact, sitting seems to be our most cherished activity. This suggests that the seat industry may eliminate the need for real shoes.

There are couches, recliners, lounge chairs, divans, high chairs, low ones, folding chairs, benches and an endless variety of automobile seats, as comfortable as any hide-a-bed. That's why athletic shoes or sneakers are in solid. They're big, ugly, comfortable footwear designed for exercise or house slippers when you're resting.

We seem to begrudgingly move from one seat to another—the kitchen chair, to the living room seat, to the car seat, to the office swivel chair, to the nice eat and rest lunch seat. This lunch seat may also be a car seat if you're one of thousands who line up, engine running while waiting in your car to order some fast food. Again, about the only movement necessary comes from your mouth—another real paradox, since the relentless marketing of technology (TV, computer games etc.) has discouraged social mouth movements at home.

Those of you who still walk may have noticed this line of cars with passengers conserving their energy as they await food unnecessary for their survival or health. I have. Approaching a Jack-in-The-Box on foot for a monthly grease fix, I saw a long line of cars rumbling in wait to order food. No human movement. Assuming the inside must be crowded, I was astounded to find no one at the counter but a bored-looking employee.

"Where's the lunch crowd?" I asked after ordering some fries.

She smiled. "They're in their cars, but it's much quicker when they come in and order."

Twenty-First Century society is teeming with anti-exercise and anti-nutrition marketing strategies that may not be aware of their "anti" health messages. Maybe they don't care. It doesn't really matter. We relentlessly and naively conform to the marketing messages by adapting our behaviors to less activity. The more comfort, the less energy we burn, *the better off we are.* But remember, we are what we do, and the marketing message tells us eating a lot and doing less is fine.

☙ ❧

Must sound convincing since so many of us have adjusted to this over-indulgent, comfort-laden lifestyle. As an added mockery of independent thinking, there's an incredible paradox to the multibillion-dollar comfort marketing success. It's the multibillion-dollar expansion of the counter comfort industry. It's the marketers who help us compensate for our sluggish lives with a wide assortment of dieting and exercise programs. Marketer "A" makes plenty of money getting us *fat*, while Marketer "B," who may still be Marketer "A" in disguise, makes plenty of money by preaching *thin.*

The marketing business has it both ways. You don't have to walk when you can sit comfortably watching TV. There are treadmills for walking. The only losers are the duped consumers who are learning that walking is exercise only when part of an expensive athletic club program.

Here's an example of how marketing has changed walking (the activity) into walking (the exercise). The people in that car you noticed circling the block were looking for a parking place close to the gym. There they'll mount a great moneymaker called a treadmill and walk without going anywhere. On a pleasant, sunny day in San Francisco, I saw such a phenomenon unfold. Two young women parked their car in front of a fitness gym after circling the block twice. In about five minutes, the same two women could be seen, through huge gym windows, walking to nowhere on those expensive contraptions called treadmills.

Walking on a treadmill is literally interacting with the wonders of life—on a treadmill. You're going nowhere which is becoming the quintessence of urban life—going lock step to nowhere on a treadmill.

Although, admittedly, I don't personally know most of my readers, I wager each one has somewhere to walk that is infinitely more interesting, educational and exciting than a walk to nowhere on a treadmill!

But, "Gee whillikers," you argue, "what about when there's ten feet of snow on the ground or 120° of heat?"

Well, if you're not into snowshoes or saunas, there are still a zillion treadmill options in life. For me, that's when Richard Simmons has all kinds of fun tapes to follow, especially for seniors (see the appendix). Or, how about learning a few dance steps, walking around an indoor museum or shopping mall, thoroughly cleaning your house or jumping rope. Then again, you could shovel snow, get up to change TV channels or wiggle your ears. Any activity burns calories, impedes muscle loss and sure beats relying on marketing fitness contraptions.

Also, don't forget one more earth-shaking paradox: Using a treadmill requires preparation, like going to a health club or your basement, etc., while actually walking "to" a treadmill to walk "on" the treadmill doesn't.

Treadmills are fine for medically monitoring vital signs under controlled energy output. Seems, however, like that is just a once a year activity and it's not free.

There's another common activity that's been transformed into exercise by the fitness marketing industry. It's one of treadmill's cousins that train you how to "step up" to better fitness. It's become a packaged aerobic step exercise with an adjustable plastic contraption that kind of looks like a step. Well, here's an innovative breakthrough suggestion. Try taking more stairs and fewer elevators and escalators, as a great—and free—muscle strengthening, calorie-burning activity/exercise.

As a supplement to walking outdoors in extreme weather, treadmills may have a place, in addition to their medical uses. Otherwise, P.T. Barnum's sucker comment was a glaring understatement.

We tend to believe the sales pitch because it seems sooo good. It promises a more comfortably inactive lifestyle. Don't worry about your sagging muscle tissue, that's what fitness programs are for. Not convinced of marketing's "get fat—get thin" paradox? Then review the financial gains for marketers. Convenience technology charges thousands of dollars to perpetuate your languid lifestyle, before exercise marketers come to your rescue.

As an example of the power of marketing, treadmills are one of the hot items in the new millennium. In "The Best of Fitness Equipment" section of the Jan/Feb. 2005 issue of *HEALTH,* there's the "Life Fitness T9i" for $5,500. It's a treadmill that does everything but walk for you. Or, for $3,000 you can ride a bike in your living room, while enjoying a virtual reality scenic tour. How about rowing without the water? Just $850 for a "Concept 2 Indoor Rower Model D."

One of those steps that lead to nowhere is cheaper still. If the "STAIR" fulfills even one of its marketing comments on the box, it would be worth ten times as much as the retail price of $44.99. It offers a way to "firm all muscle groups—develop a beautiful body. High-intensity, low impact aerobic/cardio exercise. Burns more calories than walking in less time." If you can't find real stairs, there are plenty of these "steps" on the market.

A lot of these apparatus are available in your local gym or athletic club. Of course, you're also paying a pricey fee for the facilities and their fitness programs to offset your sluggish lifestyle.

An added sad commentary on today's marketing was a report on national news as recent as March 27, 2005. It was about a gym with small apparatus for little pudgy kids who want to lose weight. The implication was some kind of major breakthrough for kids, while nothing was mentioned about simply changing their pudgy lifestyles! All of us are driven by habits we develop from our cultural interactions and observations. And, if we simply developed the habit of remaining active with frequent walks, and all sorts of movements wherever we are (even fidgeting) we'll feel better, stay healthier and trimmer—promise!

We are what we do, and it is becoming increasingly apparent that we're not really doing much with our *matter*. We are a nation of spectators with an acquired taste for "virtual reality." We cheer our teams as if we were out there performing with them. In reality, most of us are sitting somewhere, watching, while stuffing our faces and downing a few beers. We barely move, other than our mouths. We watch everything from competitive sports, to perpetual sitcoms, to musicals, to adventure tours where people actually walk. To restrict our movements further, technology has given us remote controls. It's no longer necessary to leave your seat and cross the room to change a channel or station. Any wonder why we are becoming a nation of fatsos?

Alarmingly, that muscle between our ears is also being seriously neglected. Watching TV and other spectator activities aren't really activities in the sense of doing something. The brain needs exercise or it atrophies like any other neurochemical tissue. Passively being entertained does nothing to enhance your brain, fitness or health. The human body wasn't ingeniously created for a passive, sybaritic life of disuse.

Charles Darwin's principles of natural selection posit a grim picture of our future if we continue to do less, while expecting more.

☙ ❧

Here are a few other well-researched findings that aren't common knowledge. If you want to enhance your mood—exercise! If you want a free, non-prescription pain killer—exercise! If you want a free narcotic with no side effects—exercise!

It's not too good to be true; it's just a well kept secret. The hormonal chemicals are called endorphins and enkephalins. They're naturally occurring endogenous proteins that activate with analgesic effects similar to morphine. I'll bet virtually all readers are aware of morphine sulfate. It's about the best analgesic on the market (or street) with mood elevating, euphoric producing feelings that can also serve as stress reducers. If you want to know how you can get it, you already have plenty of it. This natural narcotic is just waiting to be summoned. And, of course, the magic catalyst is exercise, aka activity.

This phenomenon is no secret to athletes who frequently experience feelings of euphoria or analgesia during physical sports activities. I've lost count of the times during my youth when I entered the locker room after a football game with broken nose, lacerated brows or lips, while feeling great with no pain. So add these findings to your list of exercise benefits. Sorry, a walk around the block or four push ups won't give you a euphoric high. But if that's more than you've done before, it's a great start that will sure give you a lift.

Another conclusion, backed by numerous studies, is that the lack of exercise exacerbates problems of old age, including mental deterioration.

There are simply no negative side effects to physical activity, regardless of your age. That's unless you believe feeling and sleeping better, being healthier, trimmer, sharper, clearer thinking and more self-reliant are downsides.

But don't confuse exercise with the "workouts" at your local fitness center. It's apples and oranges. Going to the gym a few times a week is fine for the young studs and body builders, while leading an active life remains essential for both health and fitness. Occasionally "pumping iron" in the local fitness club won't keep you fit, an active lifestyle will.

Seniors, please pay special attention to these recent research findings. Too many old people believe walking may increase the probability of a hip fracture because they fall easier when walking. Just the opposite occurs. Continued walking into old age preserves "strength and balance" which reduces falling. To all my senior peers: Walking for seniors, regardless of age, is a genuine panacea that will work to preserve your mind and body. In fact, the more active your life, even while at home, the more fit and healthy you'll remain. Disuse is everyone's major health enemy.

଼ ଼

If a picture is worth a thousand words, a "Homunculus" speaks volumes about our future physiology. You may recall, from high school, some of those basic physical science textbooks showing this strange little guy, called a Homunculus, representing different physiological processes through anatomical exaggerations. The little guy in this book also has restructured anatomy to point out how persistent changes in what we do could affect our bodies.

Working upwards from the lower extremities, the legs of the Twenty-Second Century Homunculus would have atrophied considerably, since people by then would be thoroughly accustomed to spending most of their time relaxing in some sort of a seat. Resting on those seats, a small, tight, muscular posterior would be unnecessary and uncomfortable. Hence, a nice, fat, pear-shaped bottom. The arms and hands would be further re-proportioned, with the arms mainly used as handles to keep the well-used hands and keyboard fingers attached to the body. Fixated on TV and computer screens, bulging eyed myopia would represent normal vision.

Marked changes in brain behavior relations would tend to compromise the size and spherical shape of the cranium, the brain's container. Exceptionally adept at processing verbal information and analyzing data, the Twenty-Second Century left hemisphere would flourish. The right hemisphere's more intuitive efficiency processing visual, spatial relations (including street savvy) would tend to atrophy. The front of the brain, frontal lobes, concerned with much of our humanness, such as a sense of humor and caring for each other, would also probably shrink. Who needs humans for company when you have all those electronics?

The Twenty-Second Century Homunculus is now complete. Spindly legs, huge belly, fleshy tush, enormous muscular fingers attached to frail bony arms, bulging eyes and a weird shaped head. Below is a sneak preview of what a sight we would be. Take a good look.

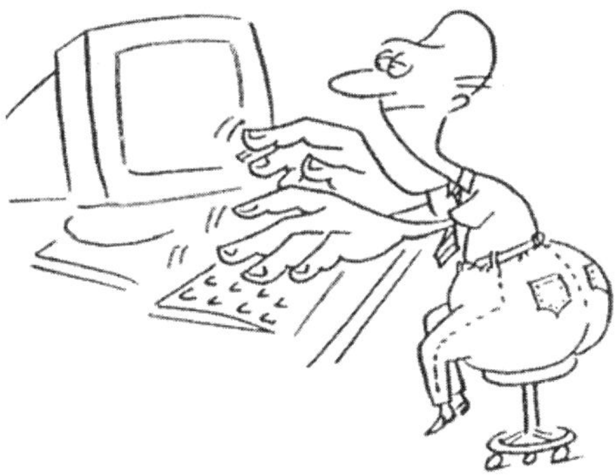

TWENTY-SECOND CENTURY MAN
"Homunculus"

Fact Summary

1. You *really* are what you do.
2. Americans, especially urbanites, keep doing less—except for eating.
3. Technology marketing is convincingly selling comfort and inactivity at the expense of fitness and health.

4. To counteract the multibillion-dollar comfort market, a multibillion-dollar diet and fitness market has emerged with band-aid solutions to serious problems.
5. Marketers of apparatus define walking as a treadmill exercise.

CHAPTER 9

What Matters Is You

As a species, we are so much alike that even the most discerning Martian wouldn't be able to tell us apart. It doesn't matter where we were raised or whether we were fallopian tubed or test tubed into the world. Either way, what a miracle we are.

We look so much alike, with sparse body hair clustered in peculiar places, and a skin of various hues and shades, yet we're defenseless against extreme temperatures while generally impervious to deadly bacteria. We walk upright with a gait that can only be described as human.

Our structural engineering permits delicate facial contortions that appear in subtle variations as smiles, laughs and frowns, those universal messages we all understand. Our hands are also exquisitely engineered to thread the smallest needle or lift twice our weight.

Beneath our skin we are still alike. There's a neuro-anatomical network of cells, bones, vessels and tissue, all working in unison to keep us alive and moving in the same evolutionary direction.

You may have noticed that Part I was all about the species—you, not the, ah, you-you, the individual. Indeed we're all alike, yet more astonishing, each of us, as an individual, is a unique creation.

There are over six billion of us, and we are as different from one another as our fingerprints or DNA. One more reminder of what a miracle we truly are.

So, for the rest of this book, you're the only individual that counts. It's time to turn away from the six billion and focus on number one—you.

Knowing your allies and enemies, how you function as a species and what's nutritiously good and bad for you isn't enough. It's vital you understand your own personal, unique strengths and weaknesses. That insight is your first line of defense against poor health and retarded fitness.

A redundant, but necessary warning throughout this book is to not take yourself for granted. Once you've succumbed to such folly, you simply get used to bad habits and those sprouting symptoms of wilting health. That's when being fat is no longer a problem, it's just a bigger you. When driving everywhere rather than walking anywhere is a fact of modern life, and when labored breathing after that thirty foot jog from your house to your car is, well, no problem.

The point is, you can't improve your health and fitness unless you're aware your health and fitness need improving. Try being concerned or even aware of something that you take for granted—*duh.*

Knowing what we should never take for granted as individuals involves exploring our interwoven mind and matter. But understanding both at once might be a bit much for our minds. So we'll start Part II with the easiest first.

Which of the two is easiest to grasp is another no-brainer. Matter is the stuff scientists (and ghouls) have been examining, studying, cutting and trying to repair for centuries. We tend to forget that beneath our thin layer of skin is a complex network of fat, muscle, tendons, veins, organs, chemicals, nerves and bones, all designed to function in harmony to preserve and operate the body with maximum efficiency. There's also a something that runs the body, an energy force of some kind. This we can only describe as movement and measured by electrical impulses that disappear from instrument readouts when we die. It's also well beyond the scope of this book—or any book. So let's gratefully stay with what little we know—matter first and the mind later, in Chapter 10.

☙ ❧

As we hinted in the Prologue, since we live in an appearance-oriented society, our first step is to take another good, objective look at ourselves. A full-length mirror, a scale and a few simple calculations suffice as our "pay attention kit."

If a mirror isn't handy, just stand up straight, tilt your head downward without leaning forward, and see if you are looking at your belt, knees, your shoes or just your belly. Then, on either side of your belly are varying degrees of protrusions called external oblique muscles or love handles. Between your thumb and index finger, grab about an inch of skin surrounding one of the two areas and squeeze lightly. See if the captive flesh is thicker than one of those juicy smoked sausages.

Now try to calculate your *Body Mass Index* (BMI). It's much more than a number. It's a digital alarm that compares your score with nationally standardized tables that translate into health risks for diabetes, heart disease and other medical ailments.

Try this simple version, and if it's too complicated, ask your neighbor's kid or your eight-year-old daughter for help with the math. Most kids today have a calculator in their backpack. You simply record your weight in pounds and height in inches. Then square the height by multiplying your height by your height. Now divide your weight by your squared height. Finally, multiply your answer by 703 and you'll have your official Body Mass Index to jar your complacency.

Here's an example to follow with a 165 pound, 73 inch man.

a. Square the height: 73 X 73 = 5,329
b. Divide weight by the squared height: 165 divided by 5,329 = .0309
c. Multiply the quotient, .0309, by the constant (703): .0309 X 703 = 21.72.

That man's BMI of 21.72 is well within the healthy range for anyone, including 75-year-olds. That geezer happens to be me (or I). With an active lifestyle, no special diets, fitness clubs or apparatus, just me. The secret formula is simple. I practice what I preach.

In the Appendix, Section B, there's a slightly more complicated BMI formulae for the math wizards and Europeans. It uses meters instead of our U.S. inches, and kilos for pounds. The Appendix also provides some useful interpretations of BMI scores. For example, scores of 20 to 24 are in the normal range, 25 to 29 is overweight, and over 30 is obese. You might as well try the simpler equation first. Although the number is a little less accurate, its meaning is no less significant.

If you prefer charts or hate equations, Section A in the Appendix is all you need to work out and understand your Body Mass Index. You may be wondering, *Why the hell didn't he tell me that in the first place?* Sorry! I thought you might like to exercise your brain a little.

At this point in your self-examination of what you are as an individual, take another peek at the mirrored you. If your belly blocks the view of your feet, if your lightly squeezed love handles are thicker than Kielbasa sausage, or your BMI is in the high twenties—you might consider taking your health, your fitness and your life more seriously, less for granted. For starters, you're probably eating too much and exercising too little.

While you're at it, try to separate the real you from those stereotypes that too easily lump you into a category like pretty or ugly. Those terms try to define your social worth, not your health. The NFL may put a positive spin on the excess weight of huge linemen even though fat is still unhealthy. Then there's the other extreme—when being too thin is both a serious medical problem and a model's major asset. Hopefully you're none of the above. You just want to keep fit and healthy. So keep reading.

While your mirror watches you, begin to move a bit. Are the motions youthful, effortless? Is the posture sagging old and heavy, or light, vibrant? These are more symptoms of the state of your good health and fitness that add to your personal portrait.

Body movements provide valuable clues regarding the fitness of your muscles. Although increasingly debatable in our armchair society, our leg muscles still tend to get more strenuous exercise than other muscles, especially if we're overweight. A 5′10″ 142-pounder will practically fly up those eight stairs while Mr. Five Foot Ten at 215 pounds would be packing an extra 73 pounds up that formidable stairway to Everest. There are other mini activities you do most every day—like putting on your socks. Instead of taking it for granted, observe your movements carefully. As you grasp a sock and lean toward your feet, is it an effortless reach, or a snap, crackle and grunt? Think about it.

Flex one of your calf muscles (lift a heel as if you're about to walk). Unless you don't do walking, the calf muscle will feel considerably harder than when relaxed. In other words, your calf muscles are being used. Now flex your bicep (that's the muscle on top of your upper arm.) If you don't know how to flex it, try picking up a chair with one hand, palm up while feeling the hardness of the muscle with the other hand. If there's no difference in its size or density when flexed or relaxed—no wonder you didn't know how to flex the bicep. You probably forgot how to use it, and it's another of those health and fitness facts. If you don't use them (muscles) you'll lose them.

ଓ ଛ

Taking a serious, objective assessment of your matter should also include a second opinion by a physician—the first opinion is reserved for you. While you're at it, keep a record of your pulse and blood pressure to facilitate your physical exam.

"But that's the doctor's job," you may argue.

Wrong! The major responsibility for your health is your job.

Blood pressure is occasionally forgotten by your physician, or your uneasiness in the physician's office can cause an unusually high blood pressure reading. If you can't afford a $50 digital blood pressure kit, many drug stores have one set up at a table for free. Your physician should know about your typical blood pressure readings to offset either his forgetfulness or your one time pathologically high reading (because of your nervousness about going to the doctor.) Although high and low blood pressure is an individual thing, Section C in the Appendix gives you some baseline parameters.

You are better qualified than a physician to examine your body because it's your body, not the physician's. You see your flesh daily, not just once every six months or yearly. Only you can easily detect even gradual changes in your body, like fatter thighs, a new mole, tighter pants or unusual sensations. You are your first line of defense against poor health—provided you pay attention and stop taking yourself for granted.

Your physician is no more or less wise, well adjusted or human than you. She needs to know from you about changes you've observed, where it hurts or if the pills you're taking are working. Obviously your physician doesn't know what's bothering you or where, unless you tell her. Otherwise medicine has to do it the slow, methodical way until one of the prescribed tests or procedures are not "normal." You could have been a great help if you knew your body. It would not only save the physician a lot of time, she would be more inclined to examine you as an individual than a norm (the medical profiles of most healthy persons).

Physicians today don't have much time for small talk, so when they ask, "How are you today?" "What brings you here?" or "What's the problem?" don't be coy—be direct and honest. Write down your concerns and medical questions before the exam. Don't deny your physician the privilege of working for her salary. You are the customer and it's your body! Even if you feel fine, a yearly physical examination is an important health and fitness alarm system to alert you to possible subtle chemical or tissue changes requiring treatment.

While you're at it, have your physician check your calorie requirements. Calories represent the amount of heat releasing energy necessary for your body to work normally. What you eat contains fat, carbohydrates and protein. Each of these components stores a different number of calories per gram. Excess calories, i.e. beyond needed for basic energy needs, are unfortunately stored as body fat. If you're active, however, you needn't be particularly alarmed. The more active you are, the more calories required to burn for energy. The problem is, when you have calories "to burn" and you're not burning them. It's a simple equation: unused calories equal fat. As a quick example of calorie needs, exercise-driven athletes need at least 2,800 calories per day, while slugs require about 1,600 calories.

Blood tests, heart sounds, chemical balances can reveal all sorts of medical evidence that something isn't right—for the average person. That person, of course, is not you, which is why scientists of all disciplines embrace the idea of false negatives and false positives. False negatives can be a nightmare when your physician tells you your tests results were fine (negative) even though you're not. False positives are just the opposite. The lab results tell you, through your physician, that the cancer test was positive when, oops, it's not. Those mistaken results bounce you from the floor to the roof—Yikes!

There's no hidden message here, just a few more reminders of your foremost responsibility. Check your body often as your first line of defense against poor health and fitness. As a second line of defense, see a physician once a year and if results cause a stomach freefall, get a third opinion. False positives are cruel, false negatives are deadly, and individuals like you aren't the same as medical averages.

Here's a personal example. Since my 20's I've had a prostate gland the size of a baseball. Such a little monster chokes the urethra (the urine tube from the bladder) causing all kinds of urinary problems like the bladder infections of prostatitis. Fifty years later there's a prostate specific antigen (PSA) test for prostate cancer. Although it can accurately announce the bad news for many men who may have cancer, it also announces the bad news for many men who are cancer free. Like them, for me it's a pain-in-the-neck false positive. So, don't forget that third opinion.

Incidentally, my last urologist was a competent physician with a caring bedside manner, yet even the best physicians can occasionally overlook individual differences in their clients. That's the time he prescribed a beta-blocker medication that he professionally concluded might reduce the size of my prostate gland. "Worth a try," I agreed. The next day, after popping one pill, I was so weak I could barely get out of bed. My friend, the physician, hadn't taken my blood pressure, which is characteristically low normal. I was also unaware that this particular pill is a hypertension medication that drastically lowers blood pressure.

Physicians are just fallible humans like the rest of us, and as long as they act like humans, I forgive them—he seriously apologized.

One last tip for this chapter, if you follow these pretty simplistic suggestions to knowing your matter, you'll take better care of yourself without even trying. Promise.

Fact Summary:

1. Minding your matter begins with becoming thoroughly acquainted with your body. There's no other exactly like it.

2. Look your body over weekly. Get to know all those inevitable positive and negative changes.
3. Get a complete physical yearly. Lab tests and a physician's stethoscope may notice something you missed.
4. If your physical is bad news, get a third opinion. You're an individual not a statistical percentage.
5. If your physical is good news (negative lab results) and you still feel lousy, get a third opinion.
6. Taking your body for granted is a prelude to both poor health and fitness.

CHAPTER 10

Mind Your Own Business

Your *Mind* is indeed your own business, and it's the most important business of your life. It's the CEO of your *Matter*. It is responsible 24/7 for your health, welfare and fitness. No vacation or weekend leisure is permitted.

Your mind has the monumental job of relentlessly directing all your voluntary activities, no matter where you are or how you feel. It's an awesome responsibility, a life long assignment. As long as you're breathing, your mind can't quit its job—it can just screw it up. Your mind may quit only when your body dies. Otherwise, no matter how hard you try to give up the most powerful leadership role in your life, you keep behaving, your body keeps on moving and without the proper guidance of your mind, life becomes a mess.

A reminder of another premise to never forget. As long as you're alive, you *cannot—not behave*. Your behavior requires about the same amount of energy regardless of the quality of its outcome. In other words, whether you engage in self-defeating bad behavior or self-enhancing good behavior—it's work, and it might as well be worthwhile. Moreover, like any successful CEO, you mustn't take your job for granted. Monitoring all aspects of your mind, while it regulates your matter, is vital in achieving your operational goals in life.

But this chapter isn't just about what you should do with your mind; it's primarily about knowing how your unique *Mind* affects your one of a kind *Matter*!

☙ ❧

Although similar to all others, your mind is as unique as a fingerprint and the undisputed power in control of your body. Your mind is a thought, a desire, a calculator, a motivator, a conscience, a planner, worrier, optimist, pessimist, self-starter, mover and shaker, bigot, zealot and caregiver. Your mind is moral, compasssionate, fearful, courageous, outrageous, lazy, disciplined…. You name the behavior and the driving force, the catalyst, is the mind.

The actions of all your friends and acquaintances are remarkably similar, yet curiously different. Each has special behavioral signatures similar to, yet different from, any other. Not too long ago I attended an athletic reunion of teammates I hadn't seen in over fifty years. Looking around the huge meeting hall at clusters of geezers, I didn't recognize anyone—until I heard the crisp, shrill, serrated laughter of Al Rubio beckoning me to my old teammates. Like so many others that evening, fifty years of wear and tear had changed their bodies, but not those mannerisms—fashioned into their persona by the mind.

Your sense of humor, mood, even your expectations are a mind thing that's uniquely you. When you burst out laughing without being physically tickled, your mind said to your funny bone, "gee whiz, that was funny," or when you cry during a movie scene, your mind told your tear ducts it was sad. Then there's the time you thought that sack was loaded with precious stones. Your mind instructed your matter to flex for the heavy lift. In surprise the sack flies over your head. It was filled with ping-pong balls.

That mind of ours orchestrates just about everything we do or don't do. So, get to know it well. We may see, hear, smell, taste or feel the same stimulus (sounds, odors, foods, etc.) as our friends; yet each of us will perceive the stimulus differently. That's the basis of the Rorschach Inkblot Test in clinical psychology.

This book obviously can't tell you about how your individual mind works. It's your mind and only you can sort that out. But you can get a pretty good idea about your mind's strategy by drawing inferences from what your body is doing. Hence, this chapter can help you learn more about how your unique mind is operating for or against the rest of you—while you decide if you're satisfied with its special, one of a kind operation.

Another reminder: Your mind is forever capable of harming or helping your body. This is reason enough for you to learn more about how your mind is affecting your body, including your weight and health.

Having mirrored your *Matter* in the last chapter, you need another mirror to reflect your *Mind.* Since your mind, intentionally or unintentionally, directs your daily activities, what you do tends to mirror your mind's leadership skills, even its hidden agenda. All you need for your initial, basic mind mirror is a pencil, paper and your memory.

Across the top of the paper list days of the week. If you're compulsive about such assignments and have a full menu of activities, you may need one page per day. Down the left side of your basic mind mirror list times, starting with when you arise and ending when you return to bed. It's not necessary to record every time you comb your hair or scratch your head. This activity list is exclusively for you in learning how your unique mind works.

Consequently, try listing all of your significant activities; let the list ferment for a while. Then look it over. You may be surprised at what you see. Like most of us, you might discover routines and rituals that unwittingly restrict your choices and conscious decisions—some sort of a relentless freight train of habits that your mind has put on automatic pilot. Maybe too many of your activities are being taken for granted. If they're necessary or healthful habits like work and exercise, that's fine. Provided that's what you want. You may, however, have lost critical awareness of other habits taken for granted. Like McDonald's four times a week or a nightly leisure of sitting at the computer for an hour, sitting by the TV for three hours, a couple of beers, and bed.

If you're in a rut, your mind is on *cruise control.* You'll recognize those behaviors by doing the same things repeatedly and without considering choices. That's a rut no less out of control than lighting a cigarette when you have one in the ashtray, snapping on the TV as soon as you arrive home, or having a dessert when you're full—because you always do.

Reviewing your activity list might also reveal the narrow boundaries and limited activities you've succumbed to over the years. There's an expansive world out there of boundless activities and experiences from which to choose, and if you're repeating the same short script, it's probably because that cruise-controlled freight train of habits has replaced the free choice of an active, independent mind.

In case you haven't gotten around to the "Twenty Values" game in Chapter 8, it's the perfect follow-up to this activity exercise.

Here's a quick refresher: List the twenty activities that you consider the most valued or cherished, even if you haven't actually done them at this point in your life. Then list the top five real or imagined activities. Now for the dollar sign ($), "P" or "S" after those activities requiring money, other persons, or a solitary experience.

What you have is an expanded fingerprint to add to your activity list. There's no other exactly like it. It mirrors your unique behavioral response to the equally unique pursuits, values, biases and attitudes in your mind—provided you're not on cruise control.

Even a cursory examination of the two exercises may provide unimaginable insights into the power of your mind over your matter.

Doing behaviorally what our mind psychologically communicates is rarely 100%. It's more like 50%. That's mainly because of how we absently adapt to what's going on or isn't going on around us. Then, before we know it, we don't know it. We just do it over and over, while not bothering to ask why. That is when much of our lives are lock step habits.

Your daily activities and Twenty Values will tell you about your conscious control over what you do, and if you are really doing what you want to do. You might even rediscover what you're missing in life. If, for example, one of your top five values is taking pictures of landscapes and sunsets, yet you haven't done it in years, what's going on? Too busy? That's a very popular and very feeble excuse, which too frequently means you simple can't break your four-hour TV habit. Too many P's behind your twenty values? P's can be negative influences if your activities surrounding them are harmful. You may need new friends with healthier values.

You get the idea. Look over your two exercises and just a bit of common sense will tell you all about who you are, where you've been and perhaps where you intend to go from here on. It's a behavioral profile of who you are as a functioning individual. A conscious reevaluation of your unconscious habits can write volumes about who you really are.

The remaining two sections of this chapter are for readers who, like most of us, aren't thoroughly confident in their feelings of self-sufficiency, self-reliance and independent coping abilities. Of course, even if you are overly confident, you're invited to continue reading the remainder of this chapter if you're curious about what you don't need to read.

☙ ❧

Here's another scientific fact to assist you in better knowing your precious, one of a kind mind and matter. Perceived stress hurts your body and can markedly reduce your activity rate. Since the focus of Part III of this book is about you as an individual, the term perceived is important. It's your personal view of what you consider stressful. It could be anything from the destruction of your home, loss of a loved one, job pressure, marital problems or the guy who takes the parking place you were waiting for.

Perception, like beauty, is always in the eye of the beholder. One person's perceived strength is another's perceived weakness, and the same goes for stress. What bothers you may not bother someone else whose perceived stress is a cakewalk to you.

We all have our own external and internal stressors. That's no stigma by any standard. Like pain, we all experience it in perceptively different ways. Also, like pain, prolonged stress can beat up our matter and plunge any of us into depression, which is another way to hurt our bodies.

Chronic stress and resultant low moods are dealt with in a variety of ways. One popular negative approach is over eating, another is brooding inactivity. All of these findings have been well researched, and offer a powerful suggestion that stress reduction techniques belong in this health and fitness book. Why? Because unwholesome, unhealthy lifestyles are physically and mentally stressful, while conversely, stress can cause unhealthy lifestyles.

If medication crosses your mind, think *last resort*. If they work at all, pills typically mask stress symptoms; they don't deal with the underlying problems. Another caution: medications usually have negative side effects—plenty of them.

Like so many other problems in our lives, being aware of our unique stressors and coping mechanisms is a good start toward stress management. You might be gnawing on the slight possibility that you're in a bit of a rut. Wouldn't it be nice to change some of your lock step habits in pursuit of more fulfilling activities? Besides, you may note, you're a tad heavier than you should be and exercise isn't part of your present routine.

Here's a sidebar preface to the next chapter. Obesity can be as symptomatic of stress as alcoholism or drug abuse. That's why our Bibliography includes a clinical article entitled "Relapse Prevention for Alcohol and Drug

Problems." The title could also include "For Obesity." The cravings for salt, sugar and fat by the obese are too similar to alcohol and drug cravings to ignore. They may also account for the high relapse rate of overweight persons following a rigorous diet or exercise program. Just like alcoholics, kicking a bad eating habit is virtually overwhelming if there are underlying stress related problems that haven't been addressed. Avoiding sugar-rich foods by the hooked really isn't much different from the abstinence struggle of the alcoholic, and all too frequently just tackling the symptom won't cut it—for long. This is especially true if the alcoholic hangs out with other heavy drinkers or the obese who hangs with other inactive, heavy eaters.

The actual therapeutic intervention in this paper is a "cognitive-behavioral model" that begins by helping readers explore all the high-risk situations contributing to relapse, like the glutinous friends of a struggling dieter.

This treatment approach is included as a reminder that overeating and under exercising can be symptomatic of much more than being a slug with a big appetite. So, if you're one of those individuals who can't figure out what keeps pulling you back to a soft couch, loaded with fries and burgers, don't stop now, keep reading at least until you finish Chapter 11.

One more self-assessment exercise may help you further sort out whether or not your mind is satisfied with your body, or if there's more than your share of stress in your life.

Under Section G in the Appendix, is a Stress Questionnaire. If you're still curious about what's prompting some of your self-defeating behavior, completing this questionnaire might be helpful. Read the instructions carefully, then read each of the 22 items, and on a separate piece of paper, record your opinion of each item. Remember, a "1" means you absolutely disagree, while a "5" means you completely agree.

A. Add up the 22 numbers reflecting your opinions. Wait, don't get excited, your total score doesn't mean much. All by itself it has no statistical validity. Statisticians call such a number raw data. It is not a magic number informing you of you present stress level or just how stressed out your really are. If, however, your total is over 110, you might have flunked arithmetic in grade school, since the maximum raw score is 110. On the other hand, if your total score is exactly or around 110, you're no doubt a Pollyanna, or just plain fibbing. At the lower end, however, with a score of 60 or below there's a high probability you don't feel too positive about your stress coping strategies. Now scan your lowest and highest items. These are official test response flags, about how you view your health, support systems and personal coping efforts. For example, if you scored a number 1 on Item 16, what are you doing about it? A psychotherapist might help.

B. Items 4, 5, 7, 8, 11, 12, 13, 16, 18 and 19 are particularly related to Frustration Tolerance. Add up these and if they are well under 30, it may suggest that whatever you're doing to minimize stress isn't working too well.

C. Items 2, 14, 21 and 22 are all about support systems in your life, and if below a subtotal of

12 you can either use a few friends or you're a contented loner, depending on your other scores.

D. Items 1, 6, 9, 10 and 17 are physical health issues and hopefully you're seeing a competent physician if your sub-score is below 15.

Again, although these numbers aren't etched in granite, if scores are significantly low, your common sense will coax you to take a closer peek at your present lifestyle, ruts and coping strategies.

Having read the last two chapters and done your homework, it's unlikely you're still taking yourself for granted. Now, you may be more keenly aware of your mind and matter than a seasoned hypochondriac, albeit less neurotic. Hopefully, you have rediscovered that only you are truly in charge of your body when using your mind. You know that taking your body for granted, with your mind on automatic pilot, heightens your opportunities for poor health, unfitness and a shortened life span. Unfortunately, in our convenience-oriented society, leading a slug's lifestyle is too often encouraged.

With a better grasp of your body's condition and your mind's power over your health, you're ready to more accurately answer some personal health questions.

Is your body's health and fitness below its potential? Is your lifestyle hurting your body? Is your mind unprepared to monitor your body's health and fitness?

If any of the answers were unequivocally yes, you're ready for some critical decision making, to be explored in the remaining chapters. Otherwise, look over the last few chapters anyway. They have plenty of worthwhile information.

Fact Summary:

1. Your Mind is the thinking, decision-making, motivational aspect of your human miracle.
2. Your Mind has the power to help or harm your health and fitness.
3. Putting your Mind in neutral leads to self-defeating ruts and bad habits—a dangerous waste of your potential.
4. Understanding your Mind's leadership role is crucial for preserving or improving you health and fitness.
5. The stresses of daily living in urban society can seriously hurt your body.
6. The first line of defense against chronic stress is better health and fitness through positive lifestyle changes. Exercise can definitely reduce pain and stress.

Part III

Know the Best Health and Fitness Strategy for You

CHAPTER 11

Health and Fitness Options

Decisions, decisions, decisions. It just dawned on me. If you thoughtfully gave unanimous no's, to those three vital questions in the last chapter on page 96, look them over again, please, one more time. Still all no's? In that case give the book to a less fortunate good friend or neighbor. You apparently don't need it or don't want to need it. Maybe you're in perfect health, perfect fitness or in perfect denial. Maybe your matter doesn't matter much—good luck. For the rest of you, with a keen self-awareness and improved understanding of those glitches in your health and fitness, you're probably interested in doing something about it. So, read on!

There are an endless variety of health and fitness interventions. It's a multizillion-dollar industry with almost as many treatments, training, diet, exercise, jazzercise, aerobic, medication and meditation options. Some are conventional, others radical, even downright controversial. There's the Boot Camp rigorous with a focus on strenuous workouts and discipline, to the Zen type gentle to the body and intense to the mind. There are all kinds of diet programs, get fit faster while feeling good spas, fitness seminars, bariatric surgery, hypnosis, warehouses full of exercise contraptions with instructtions, and a Barnes and Noble full of health and fitness books, books and more books.

ℰ𝒪 𝒞𝒮

Let's start with your health options. Without good health, your fitness becomes a low priority. Your health is the prerequisite to good fitness. Feeling sick, pained, weak, run-down or exhausted dulls the clarity of one's thinking and certainly isn't the time to focus on fitness, it's the time to get well.

Whether you are comfortable with your wellness or feeling flabby and in need of a fitness program, your first step should be that second opinion about your physical health. Remember the first opinion is always yours. Contact your family physician, HMO, PPO, Veterans' Administration, a friend's recommendation, AMA referral line or the last resort, Yellow Pages. Then get a complete medical examination to rule out any conditions that need attention or might be aggravated by a fitness regimen. Should your hired physician give you some bad news, don't forget that third opinion.

There is also that all too common psychological condition you met in Chapter 10. None of us is immune to stress, and the only medications that might help reduce stress are those "Band-Aid" antianxiety type medications. Such pills can create more problems than they solve, especially since antianxiety agents or antidepressants don't solve the underlying problem in the first place. As explained earlier, they all have side effects. So, if your earlier self-assessment led you to feel your coping strategies weren't working very well, stress might be wearing you down.

If you are still in a quandary about a lifestyle change, you may need the support and guidance of a psychotherapist or counselor. Shop around for one you can comfortably relate to. Ask friends for recommendations. Also check professional referral hot lines.

They'll typically give you several names to choose from. In the phone book these helpers in coping with life's problems are listed under social workers, counselors, psychologists and psychiatrists.

Another caveat: Don't go to your physician for the mind, other than to rule out physical concerns that are bothering your mind. He/she is your "matter doctor." They're not trained to help you with behavioral problems. Neither do they have the readiness or the time to put their medical probing on hold. In their haste or naiveté, they may give you a prescription that you certainly don't need as a first resort. Psychiatrists, medically trained specialists, are the experts in providing pills for severe mental disorders. Yet in dealing with most behavioral problems, they and their pills are also a last resort—expensive too.

These referral suggestions are included in this chapter mainly because no book or advice menu can replace an in-depth face to face chat with a professional, especially if there are no other support systems to give you a hand when needed. Got a plumbing problem and no one around to give you help? Call a plumber.

Don't forget, in urban society, stressors are everywhere, creating an epidemic of stress that rivals the seasonal flu—only year around. It's colorless, odorless and, worst of all, insidious. Under siege, your mind's protective power is weakened, your immune system is pummeled and your body's health is dangerously vulnerable. That's what stress can do to the toughest of us. Paying attention to yourself is your first line of defense, so pay attention.

Granted, there are all kinds of stress reduction cookbooks available that help kick-start you into action by exposing your denials, faults or whatever. Such books may even tweak your desire to change, however, for the chronically stressed; such books are just a good start. They're sure not the whole treatment package, so see a professional.

ᘕ ᘓ

Once you have your mind and matter in order, readiness becomes the central issue. Are you really ready to engage in a fitness program? Has your mirror convinced you of your excess weight and flabbiness? Is it worth the time, money and sacrifices necessary to commit to some sort of fitness regimen?

There are all kinds of fitness programs, and they most certainly have merit, provided you are *ready*. Otherwise none of them will work. Promise!

Readiness is everything. I learned that axiom at age fifteen. After a week of preparation, it was time to do a back flip off a small springboard. It was our ninth grade gym class, and the coach, a wise man, told me to try the back flip, only when I was ready. I really wasn't ready and not fully committed. I landed on my head. It hurt my head and my pride.

Another caveat: Don't land on your head. Wait 'til you're really, *really* ready. Then you will benefit from any fitness program and there are plenty.

Running the alphabet, there are the popular Robert Atkins diets, Deepak Chopra's more cognitive approach to health and fitness, Nicholas Perricone's twenty-eight day program, Reikian body work, Dave Tuttle's "fast" muscle building, Andrew Weil's natural approach to healing, all kinds of Yoga spin offs, and, of course, "Zap's" Gym down the street—any street.

The Bibliography lists some of the most well established diet and workout books for your consideration—if you're ready. Look them over. See how these different approaches to the same basic health and fitness problems fit your personal needs. But here is another caveat: If it sounds too good to be true, it's too good to be true.

There are simply no Twenty-First Century scientific breakthroughs that'll zing you into fitness in an effortless flash. There are no magic pills for the quick fix, no yummy diet that's really gratifying and no muscle building programs—that work while driving. In other words, none of these programs are worth the time and effort if they don't demand time and effort. They're expensive too!

If all of those regimented fitness programs, athletic clubs, special diets or surgeries require too much effort, preparation or money—you are ready for Chapter 12.

Fact Summary:

1. Make sure your health won't interfere with your fitness program.
2. Have a physical exam before taking on a diet or exercise program.
3. Stress in urban society is as common as the common cold.
4. Stress can seriously interfere with your health and fitness.
5. Health and fitness programs are big business and their effectiveness has no relation to cost.
6. Starting a fitness program before you're psychologically ready won't work.

CHAPTER 12

Get Ready To Go For It!

Every previous chapter was preparation for this one. Knowing your friends, enemies, yourself and your readiness was essential to embark upon a journey into lasting health and fitness.

It's not an ingeniously created program bursting with scientific breakthroughs. Actually, it's not a program. Nor is there anything particularly remarkable about it. That's because until recently it wasn't marketed, there are no sign-ups, and if you're not doing it, you probably didn't know about it. It's just a natural phenomenon we keep forgetting. It works better than any of the trillion "programs" out there—because its benefits are permanent, it doesn't cost money and it requires no special preparations.

Our way to lasting health and fitness is embedded in sixty years of rigorous research that wasn't really rigorous or deliberate research. It's what we scientists call Empirical Data Collection—sixty years' worth.

The experiment, or whatever, is based on years of periodic observations of a not too random sample of friends and acquaintances known since high school. A brief interview with those friends a few years ago prompted me to finally realize, *Wow, it is an experiment. It's a longitudinal study of different lifestyles.*

I confess. There was no experimental design, no controls for intervening variables, no double blinds and no null hypotheses. Just a lot of data from guys I've known for sixty years.

They were all trim, athletic, nondelinquent, fair to good students, from diverse ethnic and socioeconomic backgrounds. None of them were in poverty, and all had two parents who provided a secure, supportive family environment. Interestingly, none of the parents were conspicuously overweight. It was the pre-electronic era when TV's and cars were more of a luxury than a necessity, and computers weren't even available. It was post World War II 1940s, a period of more active, *thin* fledgling urbanites.

Keeping in touch with these guys through high school graduation, college and careers, I noticed some developmental variations in their appearances. Some were getting round and soft, while others, like me, stayed slender and firm. We were in our thirties. During the next forty years, the pudgies progressed to fatties and the slenders stayed slim. Two of the fat guys died in their fifties of heart attacks. All the trim ones are still breathing in their seventies, and only one has acquired a big belly.

Class and sports reunions provided lots of data relevant to this book. Virtually all of the fat group went from active to sedentary lives following college. This group acknowledged occasional yo-yo diets, sporadic fitness programs to compensate for their physically sluggish jobs and plenty of after work beers, computer time and TV leisure.

The slim group hadn't altered their activities much since high school except for our friend with the big belly. After knee surgery, he traded many of his outdoor activities for TV viewing, beer drinking and food orgies. Interestingly, since he was still more active than the fat group, he still looks like a slender guy, with an expanded belly.

I know, it's not much of a scientifically controlled research study, but you should realize that many of the studies you read about tend to "experimentally" exaggerate the implications of their findings.

These were "experiential" findings, which gratefully declined the smoke and mirror complications of statistical analysis. What was observed is what happened to a group of guys during sixty years of their lives. *Those who went from physically active lifestyles to passive ones got fat or died in their fifties. Those that didn't change their physically active way of life all stayed slim and firm into their contented seventies*. Not exactly an astonishing Twenty-First Century revelation, probably because there's no magic to it. It's simply active lifestyles versus passive ones. The operative term being "active."

Here are a few more facts about this sixty-year study that wasn't intended to be an actual study—more like a life long observation with conclusions.

Neither group used anabolic steroids during their youth, and none of the active group ever tried diet pills or other types of diet programs. All actives denied enrollment in any physical exercise programs, significant use of exercise contraptions or routine gym workouts. Significant use would have been anything beyond the curiosity of fooling with a device a few times.

The passive group reportedly tried all the short cut slim and trim programs from diet pills, diet meals, weight lifting and aerobic workouts, to gym exercise regimens. Some passives did the yo-yo dieting thing with up and down results, while several were periodic gym groupies as a form of workout and socializing. For them neither objective panned out. They had better luck at the bars without getting all sweaty.

Why do we now take these observations so seriously, especially since it wasn't intended to be a controlled experiment? Another no-brainer. Virtually all the current scientific research supports these sixty-year outcomes. Just review the studies in previous chapters and the Bibliography for more studies. All the conclusions are the same for women and children as well. It's a simple formula: *Eating more and exercising less is a guaranteed entree to obesity.*

These last few paragraphs provide all the clues you need to figure out what's so special about our program, that's not really a program.

So, if you're fat, flabby or out of shape, here's the million-dollar program you've been waiting for. It starts with our major premise: the only permanent way for you to stay fit and healthy is to *change your way of living*. As we promised, our strategy won't cost you money; in fact it'll probably save you a lot of money. It does, however, require the courage of independent thinking. As you probably know, this prerequisite isn't really necessary for the marketed fitness programs—provided you can afford them. It sure doesn't take any courage to pop diet pills either—if you can afford them; and it most definitely doesn't take any independent thinking to join a gym, with Jacuzzi. Marketing does the thinking for you—as long as you can afford it. It simply doesn't demand much mind power to conform to urban society's convenience-oriented values; resisting the compelling subliminal lure of marketing and technology does.

Changing your lifestyle might sound a bit unsettling at first. It means rescuing your mind from the lethargy of cruise control. Then, once you get the hang of it, you'll be able to make your own decisions and you'll be healthier than ever. As long as you liberate your mind, revamping your way of life can also be fun.

Here's an example of how resisting the ease of being stuck within the boundaries of dull routines is liberating. Below are numbers from one to nine in three evenly spaced columns and rows. Grab a sheet of blank paper, like typing paper and copy the nine-number puzzle with about a one-inch separation between all the numbers. Your copy should look like the one below, just bigger.

1	2	3
4	5	6
7	8	9

Now for the task: Without taking your pencil off the paper, draw four straight lines that intersect each of the nine numbers. If your straight lines miss a few of the numbers, try again. Give up? The diagram solution is in Section N of the Appendix.

"Hmmmm, so that's it," you lament. Moving up the numbers in a straight line from 7 to 4 to 1, the clever person who solved this puzzle pauses, prepared to turn right with a right angle and a straight line toward 2.

Then, after five tries, our clever person, who happens to be nine years old, realizes that he can't straight line all nine numbers that way. So, he bravely inches his pencil straight up the paper, beyond the 1 and the box-like boundaries set by the numbers. Having moved out of the perimeter and all alone out there, our kid sees how another straight line diving back to the right, will hit 2 and 6 dead center. Free of the boundary restrictions, our child maintains his straight line beyond 6 until a hard left begins the third straight line back to the box through numbers 9 and 8, on its way to 7. The fourth straight line is a cinch, head straight through 5 to 3.

Most adults have a tough time with this child's puzzle, principally because it requires the courage and independence to think beyond the boundaries society has created for us. Ironically, kids are much freer than adults. They haven't been hammered into submission, yet. Although, once we're adults, we're pretty much hooked, there's a cornucopia of options beyond the cloistered boundaries we have unwittingly set for ourselves. All we have to do is reclaim them, like altering our lifestyle.

Don't feel bad if you didn't solve the puzzle. I didn't either, but the lesson has been everlastingly clear. If you don't take charge of your mind, it'll be done for you, and you'll hardly know the subtle seduction ever happened—as you remain trapped in the box.

Another caveat: With your mind on automatic pilot, changing sluggish ruts won't work. You'll just grow fatter and flabbier believing in marketing's hype of comfort and convenience.

But the lifestyle changes you're about to make are much easier than you think—provided you keep thinking. All you need to start is your readiness to change and move beyond your urban, automatic boundaries of bad habits. Granted, habits, like bathing, grooming, cooking, etc., are indispensable aspects of human behavior. So keep the good ones while keeping in *mind* the following message: *Replacing the bad habits with healthful ones is one of the ultimate goals of our human behavior strategy. Your entire life involves constant human behavior, even when you don't think you're behaving—which means your behaviors might as well be healthful ones.*

Here's another essential footnote. If you believe you're too old or physically disabled to improve your health and fitness through increased activity, think again. Our strategy is for everyone—especially those who believe they're too old or decrepit to move much beyond their bedroom.

Now you're prepared for this book's final chapters of sensible changes in your lifestyle.

Fact Summary:

1. Eating more and exercising less is the primary cause of obesity and related diseases.
2. If you're fat or flabby, the only permanent way to stay fit is to change your lifestyle.
3. People with active lifestyles remain strikingly thinner than their inactive counterparts.
4. Following within the pervasive boundaries set by convenience marketing reduces your independent thinking and increases your weight.
5. As long as you stay in "cruise control" you won't change.
6. Positive lifestyle changes are for everyone.

CHAPTER 13

The Exercise Road to Fitness is a Footpath

So, here goes. We'll begin with a variety of exercises, most of which used to be called activities that you probably gave up years ago.

Each of the following exercises is incremental in that you begin by doing only what you, as an individual, can do painlessly. We start with a footpath, not a freeway. That's why our exercises are appropriate for ages 3 to 91.

To make certain our readers know how to perform every exercise, we've included photo demonstrations along with wordy explanations. We had to settle for the under 80-year-old age range, mainly because they're able to stay awake longer for photo shoots.

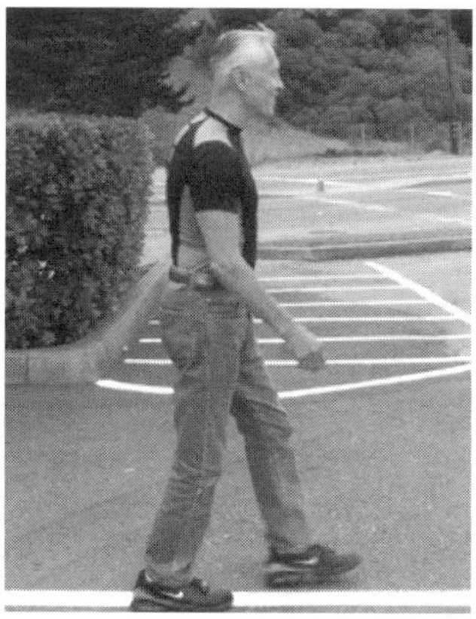

Photo 1

In Photo 1 we have 71-year-old Bob Lualhati, a good friend and indispensable collaborator in preparing this book. He's illustrating how any old geezer can handle these same exercises. In this case he's demonstrating one of our most indispensable exercises. If you're searching for a secret exercise puzzle hidden in the picture, don't bother. He's simply walking. You'll note there's no car in sight. He is also smiling, with head up, shoulders back and at a pleasant, brisk stride. Bob could continue this activity nearly forever because he's been doing it daily since age two when he crawled up the coffee table onto his feet.

Walking is much more than our most vital calorie-burning, muscle-building exercise—it can be an ever-expanding social activity. For you urbanites, your dwelling is part of a neighborhood loaded with other humans, dogs, cats, stores, homes, restaurants and parks. There's no better way to get acquainted with your neighborhood than to walk all of its streets while smiling and waving at neighbors. I promise you, your smile and waves won't go unnoticed, even by the grouch down the street; and eventually, you'll find the whole neighborhood smiling and waving back—even the grouch. It's your community, so be good to it and it will be gratefully good to you. Besides, as you get to know your neighborhood, you get fitter and healthier with every step.

Section F in the Appendix is a list of the ten best calorie-burning exercises. Notice that, mile for mile, walking is a more efficient all around activity than bicycling, and it doesn't require an expensive apparatus, a bike. Admittedly, bike riding is a good exercise. Walking is just better for a variety of reasons. You can't sit down when you walk, nor can you coast along hunched over the handlebars burning no calories.

Walking uses one-to-one gears, whereas most bikes are at least ten speeds or ten-to-one gears, which equals less work, fewer calories burned. Walking is also infinitely safer, and not everybody knows how to ride a bike.

Walking still comes out on top when compared to all other sports activities. Boxing, of course, is an excellent exercise, but it hurts when you get hit. Sailing's fine, if you can afford it and don't get seasick. Then there's all-American baseball. It's lots of fun if you don't mind either sitting around waiting for your turn at bat or standing around in the field waiting for a ball to come your way, neither of which burns calories.

How about Seadoos? Forget them! They're for macho "wannabes" who zoom around tranquil waters, making lots of noise, pollution and wakes, while burning fewer calories than grandma's walk to the store. If you love the water, try kayaking, canoes or rowboats. As for ATV's, the land version of Seadoos, they're also a "wannabe" macho man's non-exercise.

Most sports require getting somewhere to do them, while walking is the actual getting somewhere, anywhere. There's no across-town fitness center necessary. When you walk, ironically you're already in a fitness gym.

A real bonus to walking is its emotionally uplifting interaction with the outside world of people and things. Again, if you were to choose only one exercise, walking would be the most singularly beneficial to your overall health, fitness and social life. Sure, running burns even more calories. The only problem is it's too much like hard work and, for seniors, the pounding is much too hard on joints. It's also tough to say "hello" when you can't catch your breath.

Instead of a marketed workout regimen (ten bench presses, five deep knee bends in eight sets, etc.) your instructions couldn't be simpler. Walk whenever you can, as much as you can. For adults, if your trip to wherever is less than seven blocks or so and no huge grocery list—walk. Park at the far end of shopping center parking lots, grab a shopping cart and walk. When you're through with the cart, get some more exercise by walking it back to the "cart corral." Driving to Wendy's for your monthly grease fix, park in their lot, and walk inside to order. Take public transportation more frequently. It's an increased invitation to walk. By the way, have you ever noticed any fat mail carriers (except on Seinfeld)?

Dancing is a wonderful variation to walking. Line dancing, swing, waltz, salsa, folk or fox trot, it doesn't matter. They're all potential fun, a social Mecca and great exercise of additional muscles not used in straight walking.

There's an important side issue to walking as first choice for adults. While burning more calories, you burn much less fossil fuel, and we'll all be breathing less toxic pollution. Your car stays in the garage or parked in the street with the other zillion cars.

As parents, you know by now what you need to do for your children. Redirect your kids' focus from the television and computer games to the front door. Encourage outside activities, including parks, playgrounds, dog walking, paper deliveries, hula hoops, basket hoops, hopscotch, and of course, the most important, you as a walking role model. And please don't argue, "it's dangerous out there for our children." The probability of your kid being snatched off the street is about the same as winning the lottery, especially if you train your children how to survive outside in our world instead of lounging indoors.

For old folks and others with difficulties like arthritis, walking is particularly vital to your mental and physical health. Remember, use them or your muscles will get weaker, smaller, tighter, until you end up inflexibly stiff and barely able to move about. You can prevent those depressing outcomes by walking as best you can. As long as you keep trying, you will improve. Use a walker, canes, a friend's shoulder or arm. Just keep trying and smiling.

There's also a very expensive substitute to walking that marketers will be delighted to sell you. There are a variety of names for them: electric carts, electric wheelchairs, etc. Like an automobile they're guaranteed to get you around, while sitting. There seems to be more and more of these little electric vehicles silently moving about all over cities and shopping malls. This is fine for those who really need them. Unfortunately, it seems as though too many people are buying them as a first resort, rather than as a last resort. The companies that make these electric carts obviously want to sell them for their profit and your convenience—but not necessarily for your good health. Just remember, once a seat becomes a substitute for your legs, you're likely to stay sitting the rest of your life, as the few muscles you have left atrophy with disuse.

If you're able to walk very little, count the steps you take. If it's five, repeat that five over and over until five becomes six. It's a promise; there'll be no gains unless you keep trying, and the more you walk the more you gain. You'll even sleep better as you keep walking a little more each day. Remember, as bipeds, getting somewhere on foot, to the next room or next block, is walking. It is an activity so taken for granted we forget it's exercise.

If you need added incentive, there's always a four-legged health and fitness trainer. Dogs are loyal, loving friends forever and as a huge bonus, walking is their favorite activity (along with eating and sleeping). A few years ago we rescued a six year old, shaggy mutt from death row at the Animal Care and Control. He's repaid us with unimaginable treasures. His big brown eyes are two searing "happy pills" that constantly stare us into tranquil, stress reducing smiles. He's also our activity inspiration. Our walks throughout the neighborhood have tripled since he joined our family.

For those who are severely overweight, there's an unfortunate irony. One of the groups who need walking most may develop orthopedic injuries by just standing. The higher your BMI, the greater the likelihood of problems. Translated into pain per pound, overweight may mean a virtual fifty plus pound backpack of fat straining those delicate joints. The alternative is to stop walking and get fatter. Of course, preventing obesity remains vital. For the already obese, however, there are other remedies to this dilemma—besides starving yourself while sitting.

Swimming, or simply walking around in the water, is an outstanding calorie incinerator that's gentle on your joints in a relatively weightless environment. It can be an exercise Shangri-La for the obese who live near big waters, have free access to a pool or can afford pool fees. Sadly, money is always another kind of dilemma for those who don't have much of it. Should you be one of them, check with the YMCA or other community organizations that might help.

In Photo 2, it's Bob again. This time he's demonstrating one of our most popular inactivities. He's sitting, but incredibly there's no chair, seat, bench, couch or other convenient support to keep him comfortably inactive. No, the chair isn't invisible. There isn't any. He's sitting down on nothing but air. His entire back, including his lower spine, is pressed against the wall, arms hanging by his sides, palms facing the wall and both feet are flat on the floor. His knees are a few inches apart, and he is flexing and relaxing his stomach and buttocks (abdominal and glutinous) muscles.

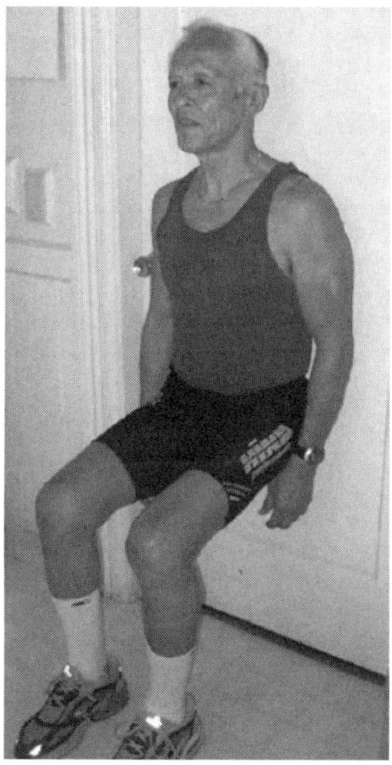

Photo 2

Isn't that a great way to rest? You can even watch TV as you strengthen the big thigh and calf muscles (quadriceps and planter flexors). You'll also be toning up your butt and stomach while the whole process burns some calories.

Just how long you maintain that position depends on what you can tolerate—plus one. Thirty seconds may seem like half an hour at first. Your thigh muscles will begin to burn and shake. Hang on to your air seat for a few more seconds. Oh boy, it'll feel so good when you finally quit.

This was one of the less excruciating, yet very beneficial, leg muscle building exercises I used to give to competitive downhill ski racers. Although they, and Lualhati, can stay "air seated" for at least five minutes, try one minute as your initial goal. For most of you that is easily achievable if you gradually increase your time, and it's really worth it. All those big muscles that keep you moving will ripple with gratitude if you include this exercise as one of your good habits. As an added bonus, all the apparatus you'll ever need for this exercise is a wall.

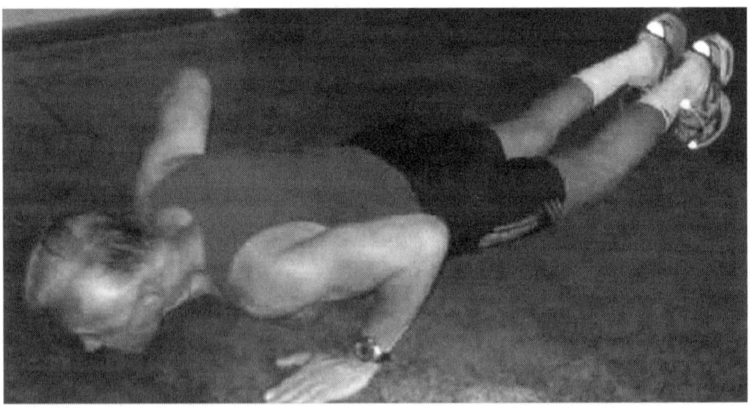

Photo 3

No, Photo 3 isn't Bob searching for his lost contact lens. He's preparing to do push-ups. Bob begins in this position because everybody from three to ninety three-plus is familiar with sleeping on their belly. As a starting point, he is demonstrating the soothing progression from a relaxed readiness to Photo 4, the top of a full push-up.

Again, there are so many in-between variations in this exercise, anyone is invited to do them at their own pace. Even an infant can do the beginning position. They just have to wait a few months before pushing their tummies off the bed. Everyone starts in the same position on their belly with arms bent on each side of the body and palms on the floor as if ready to eventually "push-up."

The ultimate goal is to keep the entire body straight as a board while pushing both flexed arms all the way up until elbows are locked, then reverse the exercise with an unflexing "push-down" until your straight body barely brushes the floor, before beginning another push-up. They can be done fast or slow and as many as you can do, plus one more. If you start with two push-ups and work up to ten—that's great. If you start at twenty and increase to twenty-five—that's great. It doesn't matter how many you do the first time. What does matter is your continued efforts to do *one more*.

It might be a struggle for persons with weak, flabby or unused shoulder and arm muscles to push their straightened body off the floor. Again, it doesn't matter. Push as much of your upper body up as far as you can, then down and up again while keeping your knees on the floor, as shown in Photo 5. As you keep trying, eventually more and more of you will rise, but only if you keep trying. Simply trying at any level will burn calories and improve fitness.

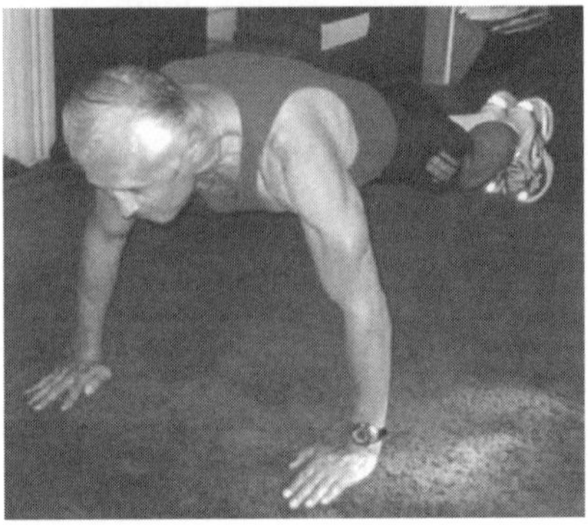

Photo 4

Photo 5 is that modified push-up position which, for beginners, is as important as one hundred push-ups for the professional athlete. It leads to toned, larger muscles, less fat and, as always, calories are burned by just trying. Push-ups are the best all around upper body exercise you can do, and require no apparatus or gym. All that's needed is a floor and your commitment.

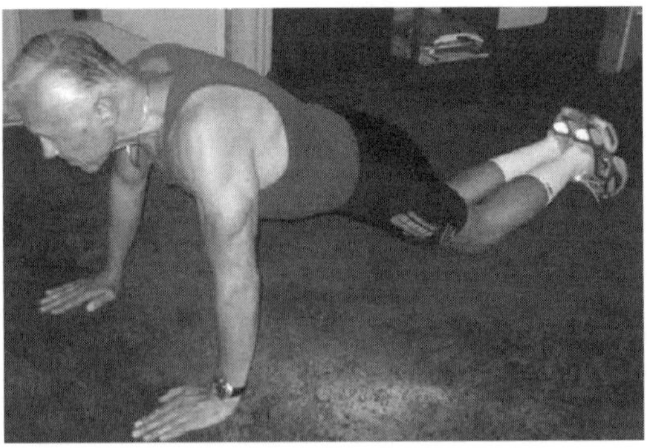

Photo 5

Take a peek at Photo 6. Is Professor Lualhati enjoying a few "Z's" after his strenuous workout or is he practicing Zen meditation? Actually neither, even though he thoroughly enjoys both. As usual, Bob's demonstrations begin with a basic position that lets everyone, from three to ninety-three-plus, know they can at least start the exercise. Photo 6 is preparation for sit-ups, an exercise as old as human history. It has probably been around for a long time because it's a good one that really works your stomach muscles.

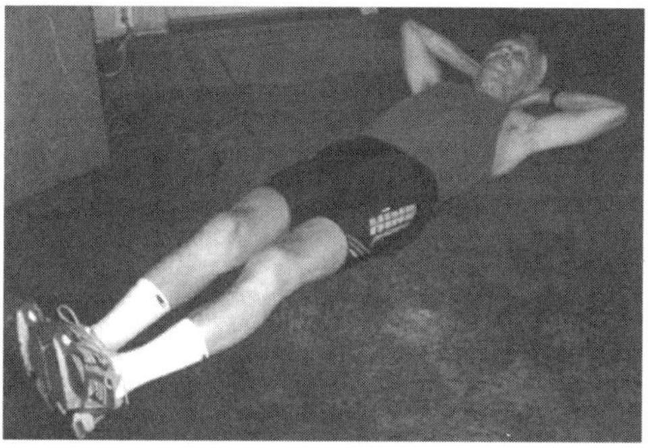

Photo 6

There are all sorts of ways to lever your upper body up from a prone position. The most difficult one, even for the athlete, is the one we're showing you first. With hands clasped behind your head, like Bob's, you literally sit up keeping your legs and back straight and heels on the floor—as a footnote, many trainers today encourage hands at the sides, rather than behind the head, as a way of preventing neck stress.

Photo 7 shows Bob just finishing the first half of the exercise. Winching your upper body off the floor flexes stomach, rump and back muscles—if you have a sturdy supply of them. If not, the only part of your anatomy off the floor will be your legs, reflexively lifting as your upper body struggles to overcome gravity.

The bad news is you need to develop those muscle fibers before "sitting up" as in Photo 7. The good news is, there are many easier ways to do a sit-up that will offer you all the muscle tension and flexion you need to loose fat, gain muscle and strength.

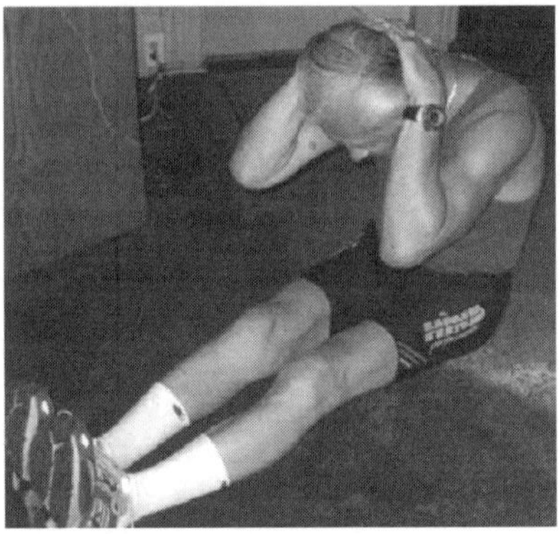

Photo 7

You don't have to be an athlete to handle the reverse of the sit-up—a sit-down. Lying on your back as in Photo 6, unfold your hands, palms down on the floor next to your waist, and push yourself up into the Photo 7 position. That's not cheating; it offers some arm muscle exercise and gets the body up into position for the "sit-down."

Now clasp your hands behind your neck, keep your back straight and slowly lower your back to the floor, while tensioning those upper body muscles to control your backward descent to the floor. Feel those stomach, back and rump muscles on the way down; even help them by trying to tense them all. It's really a good exercise that also reacquaints you with muscles you forgot you had.

If your feet fly up on the way down, have someone hold them down, or with a bend at your knees, as in Photo 8, tuck your feet under a piece of furniture. That is also a much easier way to do Photo 6 and 7 regular athletic sit-ups.

How many sit-ups or sit-downs should you do? Same as always—as many as you can, plus one!

Should the above exercise seem too tough for starters or too hard on your back muscles, the demonstration in Photo 9 is just for you.

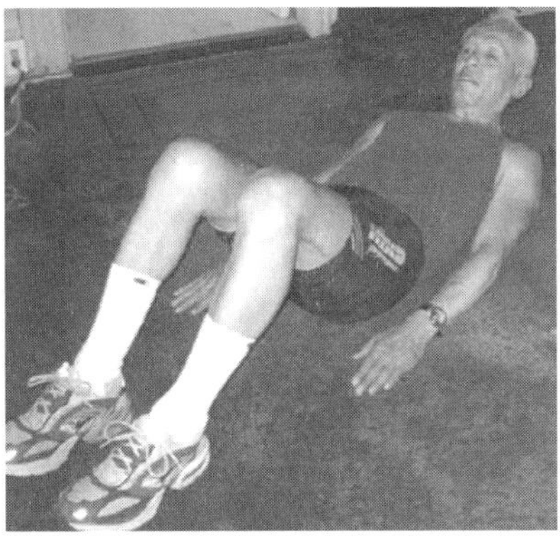

Photo 8

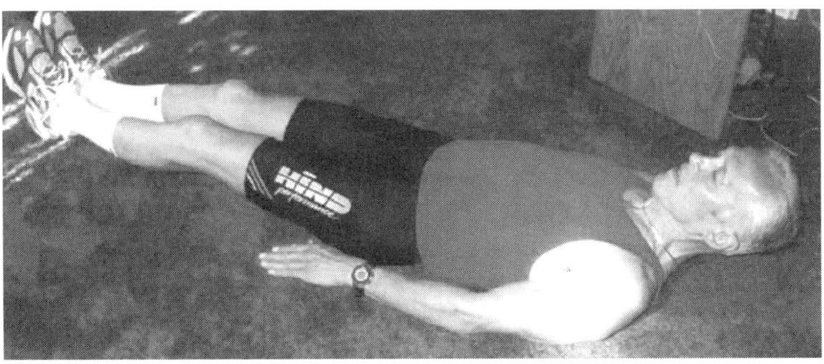

Photo 9

With arms either clasped behind the neck or extended, palms down, along your sides for support, gradually lift your straight legs about ten inches off the floor. You'll quickly feel the tension in plenty of your muscles, especially stomach muscle and some upper leg muscles. Hold the position as long as you can and ease your legs to the floor, as many times as comfortably possible, plus one.

Lualhati's position in Photo 8 is also the start of another excellent exercise for anyone who needs to effectively strengthen stomach, back and buttocks muscles without huffing and puffing their legs off the floor. Geezers love it and it's particularly helpful for tender lower back muscles.

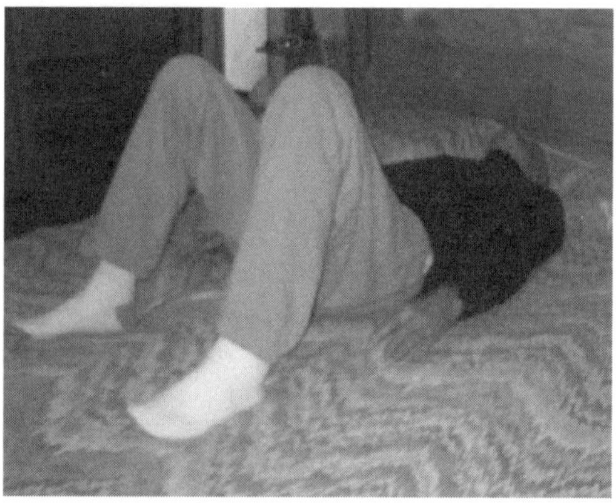

Photo 10

Photos 10 and 11 demonstrate this exercise, and you're right, that's not the headless professor in PJ's preparing for a noon nap. It's Dick Boyd, a 75-year-old friend, educator, author and one of the "active" subjects in the longitudinal study.

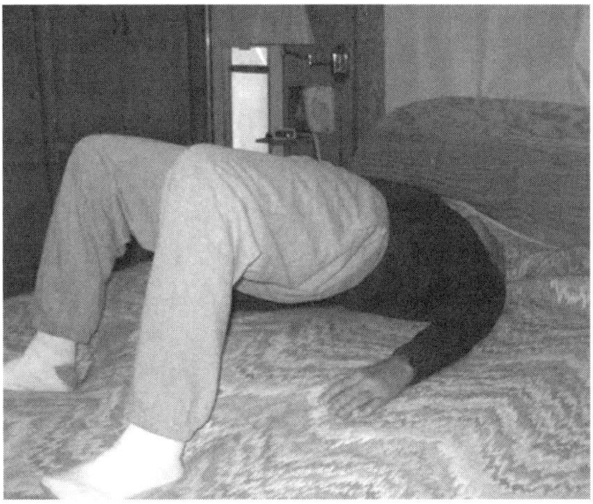

Photo 11

Although Lualhati (Photo 8) and Boyd (Photo 10) are in similar positions, Boyd chose a bed to illustrate his favorite retreat when horizontal.

Lying on your back with knees bent, hands clasped behind your neck or at your side, thrust your pelvis up toward the ceiling (Photo 11). Suspending your butt above the floor (or bed), tenses a lot of the muscles used in regular sit-ups without the hurt. You can increase the tension by pulling your navel (belly button) down toward your butt that you're also contracting. Hold your pelvis up as long as you can, plus one; then repeat as many times as tolerable—plus one. This is another very worthwhile exercise for the very young or old, provided they can stay awake.

Back to Bob Lualhati, now in Photo 12. There seems to be something in his hands. An old pair of big suspenders? Huge garters? Gigantic rubber bands? The last guess was close. Their fancy name is Flex Bands, Flex Tubing or TheraBands, which are great big rubber strips. It's the only apparatus we suggest you even try.

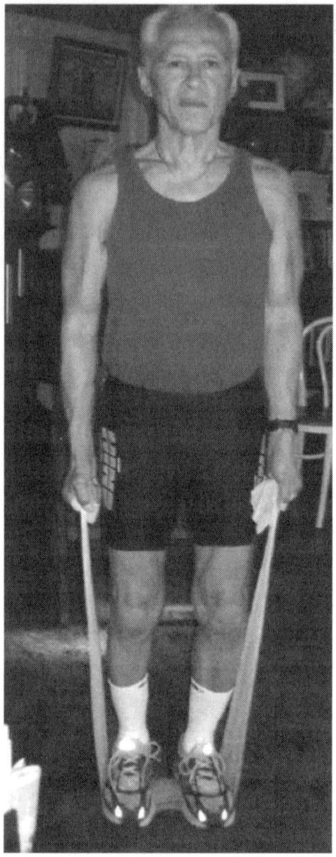

Photo 12

Here's why. When used, they are a great substitute for weights and other bigger, more expensive contraptions. They serve the same muscle building, calorie burning purpose, they utilize virtually no space in an overnight bag on trips, and they weigh a few ounces yet give the strongest athlete or the weakest geezer a keen workout to the limits of their strength and stamina. They also come in pretty colors related to thickness of the band. We all know the photos in this book are in shades of gray, so just pretend—except for the heaviest one that is actually gray.

Physical therapists, who are well trained in expanding range of motion and strengthening injured muscle fibers, have been using them for years. Orthopedic physicians regularly refer their recovering patients to physical therapists who teach them exercises that will help redevelop or strengthen atrophied muscle fiber during recovery from fractures and other injuries.

With just a little imagination and a lot of readiness to work on your flab, the exercises are endless and the big rubber strips are a fraction of the cost of gym fees, weights or those mechanical gadgets that wind up in garage sales.

In real life, their color-coding represents varying pounds of pulling tension. For example, pretend you are holding little five-pound dumbbells (representing the ends of the Flex Band) in your hands, arms at your side, palms facing out. Gripping the weights, (which are actually the ends of the Flex Bands) lift them by raising your forearms until your hands, with dumbbells reach your shoulders. Your upper arms haven't moved. That exercise is called a "curl" with five pounds of tension exerted on your muscles—mainly your biceps.

The same exercise with fifty pounders would take fifty pounds of tension per arm, which requires pretty good size biceps and very big dumbbells. So, using the ultra simple equation, T=W, the amount of muscle *tension* necessary to lift a *weight* is equal to the—ah—the weight of the weight.

Let's try that again. The amount of muscle tension in lifting any weight is equal to the pounds of the weight being lifted. Clearer?

"Sure," you say, "but don't those rubbers weigh only a few ounces?"

Sorry, you're absolutely correct in wondering how a five-pound weight is the same as a two-ounce rubber band. They're not, at least in terms of weight or appearance and our analogy isn't sound physics. We were just trying to use a unit of measure of tension that could be understood as weight in pounds. This hopefully means that if you're stretching a one-ounce rubber strip by a tension of five pounds, it is the same as lifting a five-pound weight. Get it? Please say yes!

Anyway, your knowledge of physics really isn't a prerequisite to Flex Band use. All you need to know is that, with just a few ounces of rubber you can get about the same workout at home that you would get with about five hundred pounds of weights in some sweaty gym.

Here's how, with a few examples. The thickness of these Flex Bands determines their pulling tension. Using a five-foot length of the thinnest Flex Band (which is usually yellow), grasp each end with palms out, arms at sides and let the middle of the band rest on the floor under your feet, as in Photo 12. Now, if you turn both palms outward and pull each band up to your shoulders, you are doing a curl, as in Photo 13. Incidentally, those aren't roller skates on Bob's feet nor are they little headlights. They're just funny shoes.

Doing the identical exercise (curls) with Flex Bands of varying thickness (feet still together) would require varying degrees of difficulty (pulling resistance) in curling the bands toward the shoulders. For example, the red band would require a ten-pound weight in each hand, while the thicker blue band would be equivalent to twenty-pound weights. The thickest gray band would be equal to a hefty twenty-five or thirty pound curl.

There's more! If you want heavier "weights" all you have to do is vary the length of your Flex Band by spreading your feet apart over the band. Using the lightest weight yellow Flex Band with your feet about six-inches apart would be equal to a five-pound pull in each arm. In the same position, spreading your feet further apart shortens the length of the band, while significantly increasing the muscle tension (strength, grunts) needed to curl the Flex Band.

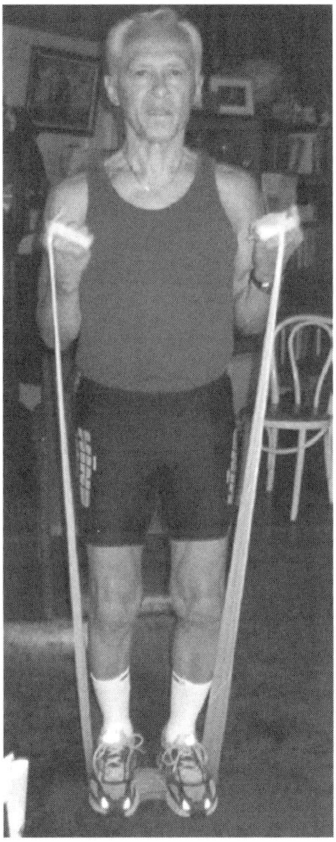

Photo 13

Back to the Professor in Photo 12. If a six-inch spread of his feet over the yellow band were equivalent to two five-pound weights, spreading his feet to twelve inches would equal using fifteen-pound weights. Had he spread his feet twenty inches apart, the Flex Band's pulling length at each end would be so short, the muscle tension in curling these shortened bands would be too much work for us. It's a simple formula: the shorter the band, the greater the tension (pulling resistance), the tougher the workout.

One hundred pounds of muscle tension in each arm would require dumbbells I could barely pick up. Anyway, the pound equivalent doesn't really matter. Just choose one of the colored strips that you can stretch with moderate effort.

Remember, if the curls are too easy, spread your feet further apart, or use a stronger band, or both. How many pounds you're pulling up is really irrelevant to your goal of gradual improvement as you do as many as you can, plus one, a couple times a day—or more. These curls are mainly (not exclusively) for your biceps.

Here's an important footnote you may have already figured out. For youngsters, who are short on strength, height and arm length, much shorter and thinner Flex Bands are necessary. Also how much of the rubber ends you grasp in each hand will shorten the band and certainly affect your difficulty in stretching the bands.

Now think about the countless variations in this exercise, and the equally countless ways you can use these Flex Bands to exercise just about every skeletal muscle in your body. All it takes is your creative imagination and determination.

For example, when you finish your curls, with arms down at your sides and palms still facing out simply rotate both palms inward toward your sides and repeat the exercise. This simple change will cause muscle tension in different parts of the forearm and upper arm including the use of less bicep, more tricep and plenty of shoulder muscles. Get it? How about a nod.

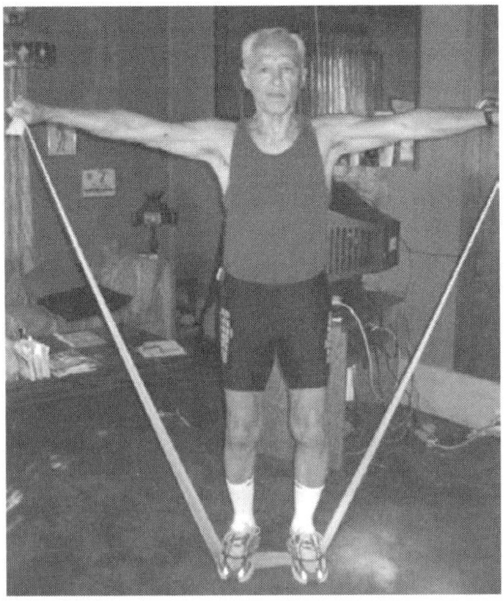

Photo 14

Photo 14 is Bob's last example, so please pay attention! Using lighter "weights" (the red ones), Bob is demonstrating a very different exercise with a similar position. Holding each red end with arms straight down, palms facing his sides, pull both arms up and out until they're nearly level with your shoulders. This is what Bob is doing in Photo 14. This exercise will help strengthen the upper back and shoulder muscles (deltoids). Variations are again awesome.

Back at your sides, if you rotate your palms another quarter turn inward so they're facing behind rather than at your sides, the same motion upwards will tense and strengthen different muscle groups in the forearms as well as the shoulder area.

Even raising both arms at varying degrees forward of the sideward raise will work other muscle groups.

These rubber exercise marvels come packaged under a variety of brand names including Flex-Band, Thera-Band, ProStretch and North Coast Exercise Band. They're all color coded to identify the pulling resistance force, some of which are scaled from 0 – 7 analogous to 7 dumbbells of varying weights.

Will these big rubber bands replace weight gyms? They may not be for the serious professional body builders like, ah, Governor Schwartsenegger. But for those who want a firmer muscle mass as well as a thinner, healthier body, those rubber strips are great!

Listen up, folks. I just remembered another fine, do it anywhere without equipment, exercise that also works the big back muscles (latissimus dorsi), shoulders, and arms. If you've ever watched Olympic gymnastics, you might have marveled at those athletes doing all kinds of exercises on "parallel bars." Maybe you remember the parallels from a high school or college gym. Even some of the more extensively equipped private gym clubs have them. No matter. You don't need those two long bars, parallel to each other (and the floor) and about five feet off the floor. One of the basic exercises was "dips." Remember? That doesn't matter either, because you can accomplish the same kind of muscle-building exercise at home, hotel room or just about anywhere there's a chair or counter top.

Photo 15 is a real geezer, who happens to be me, demonstrating a modified dip, using the edge of a chair as two parallel bars. You place your arms behind you, with the heel of each palm on the edge of a sturdy chair.

Walk your feet—followed by your legs—out in front of you as far as you can handle without wincing in pain or slipping off the chair. Keep your arms locked. Then, as in Photo 16, bend your elbows and dip down with your rump closing the gap toward the floor. Then back up to the straight-arm position. Do as many as you can plus, what? That's right—plus one. Who said you need a gym full of equipment for a complete workout?

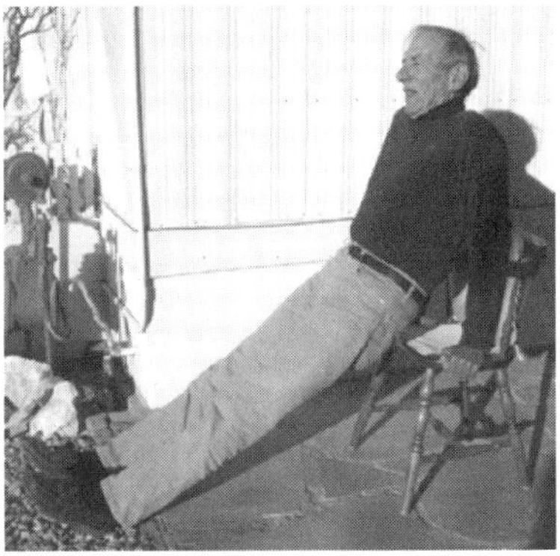

Photo 15

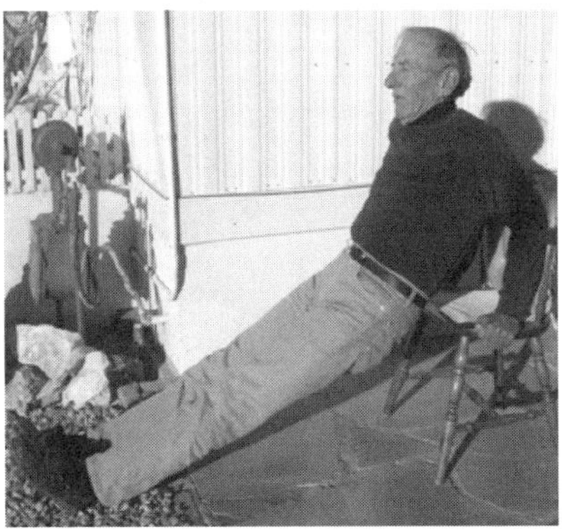

Photo 16

How could we have possibly overlooked the most precious of human genders? We didn't! We simply preserved our nurturing, loving female counterparts for the remaining photos.

Patti is a 70-something, trim female who looks 55. She's an author, mother of six, screenplay writer and, more relevant to this book, she's very active. Cheerful and engaging, Patti enjoys neighborhood strolls and rarely rides when she can walk. She also considers elevators a strange little room, crowded with people standing silently. She only uses them when her destination is beyond the fourth floor.

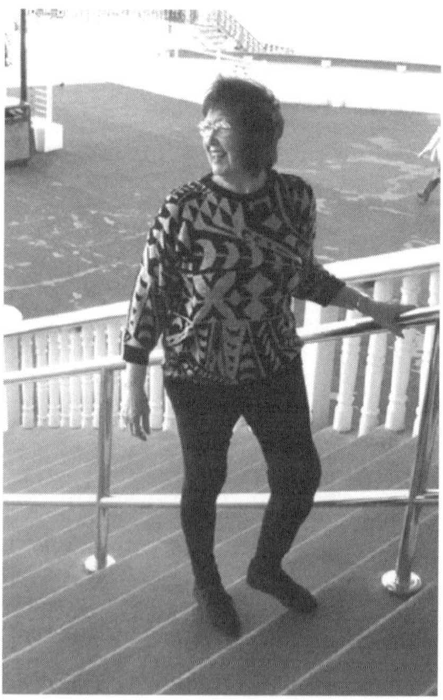

Photo 17

In Photo 17, Patti is easily climbing the 75 stairs leading to the Colorado Belle buffet in Laughlin, Nevada. She is demonstrating an activity that strengthens every lower body muscle from the stomach down, while vaporizing calories.

As we explained earlier in this book, if trudging up stairs seems like too much work, fitness marketers have skillfully converted a once healthful activity into a healthful exercise. Their logic, who needs stairs when we can sell you something that resembles stairs?

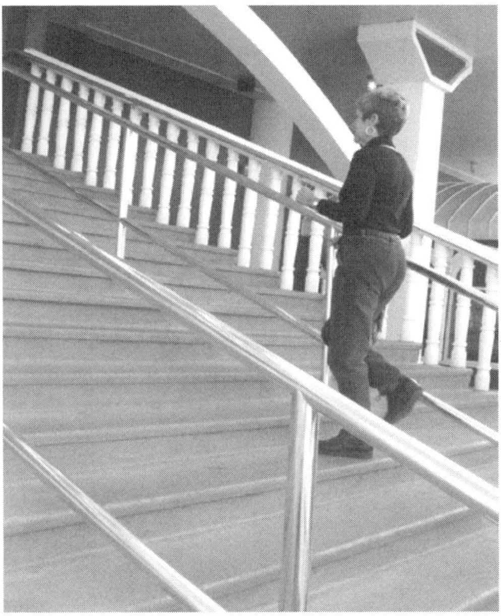

Photo 18

In Photo 18 there's Juanita, another trim stair climber, burning a few calories before dining at the Colorado Bell.

Photos 19 and 20 are demonstrations by another active senior, who still needs I.D. to obtain senior discounts. No doubt Ginger's good health and trim, young appearance has a great deal to do with her active lifestyle.

Ginger, Patti and Juanita have plenty in common. Their similarities all start with the letter "A" for activities. Activity is the general term for exercise, and Ginger also prefers calorie burning stairs to claustrophobic elevators. In Photo 19, Ginger graphically expresses her belief that stairs aren't obstacles; they're pathways to somewhere—in this case to a shrine in San Felipe, Mexico.

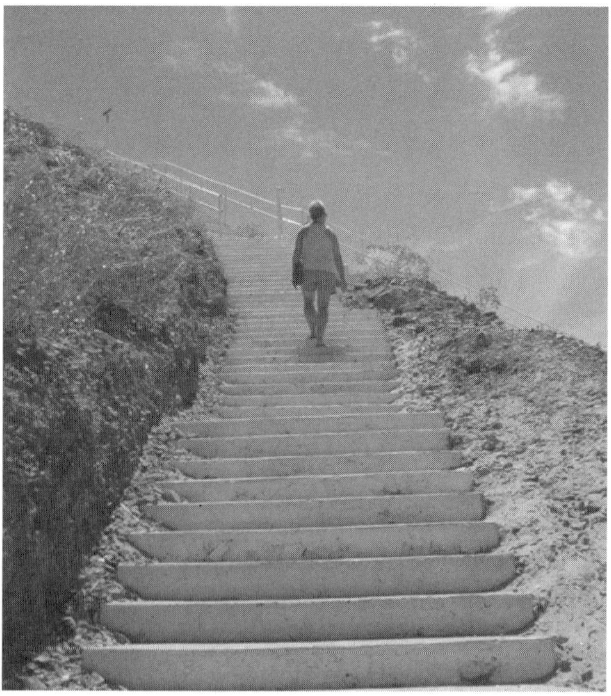

Photo 19

In addition to walking all over town, Ginger spends her leisure time caring for her garden, an activity that offers a fitness club array of exercises for free. In Photo 20, Ginger is demonstrating how a routine gardening chore is easily transformed into a healthful fitness exercise. Keeping the back relatively straight along with bended knees, she converts the back-breaking work of shoveling into a great muscle-building calorie-burner.

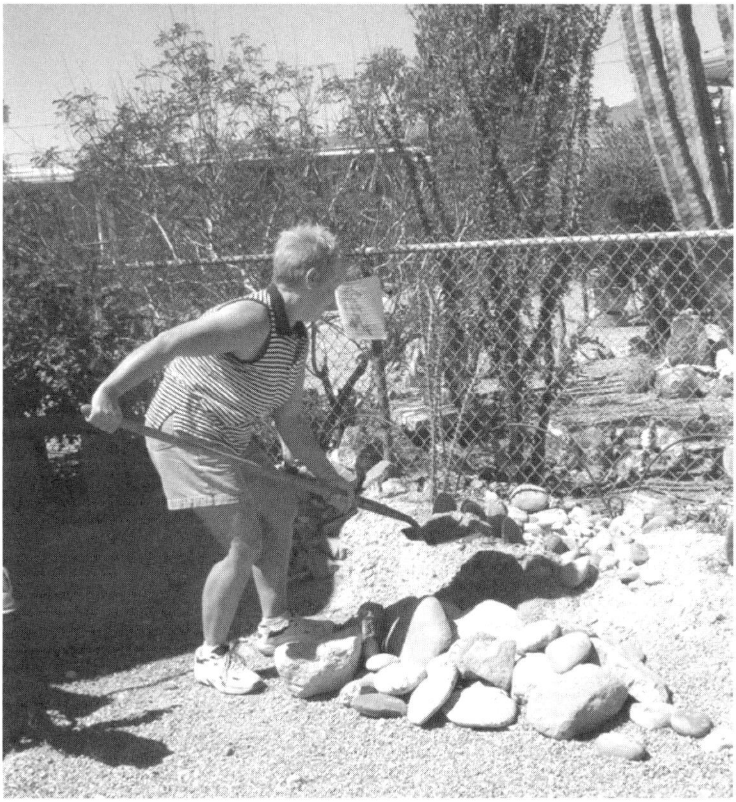

Photo 20

ꟈ ꟈ

Photo 21 combines the genders in a great workout that's also rich in social rewards. Whether it's a slow foxtrot, line dancing, swing or salsa, the payoffs in health, fitness and human contact are outstanding. Elaine and Al are happily demonstrating calorie-burning ballroom dancing.

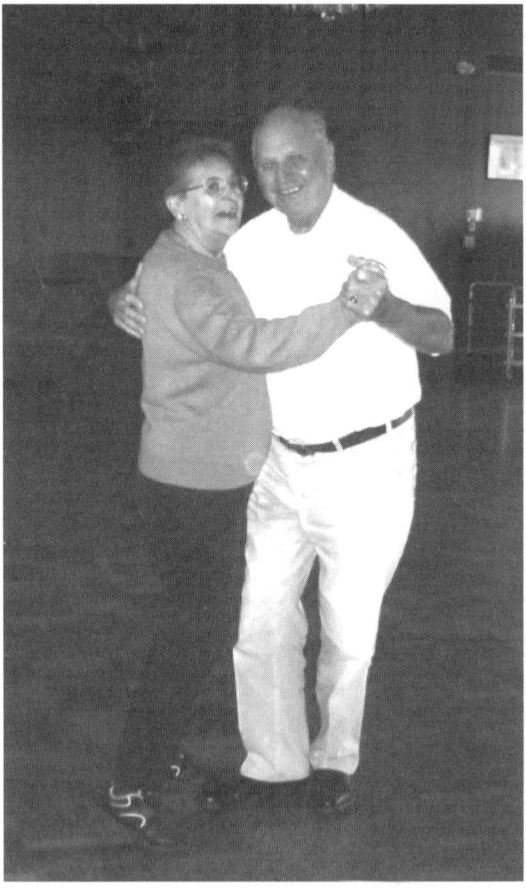

Photo 21

Finally, Photo 22 is our resident trainer, Mr. Kool. Although we technically rescued him from a last resort shelter when he was six years old, his exercise regime will no doubt prolong our lives by enhancing our health and fitness. As said earlier, thanks to Mr. Kool, the lengths of our walks have about tripled during the last four years. At age ten, he's not only an inspiration to keep moving, he's a devoted, stress reducing loyal friend.

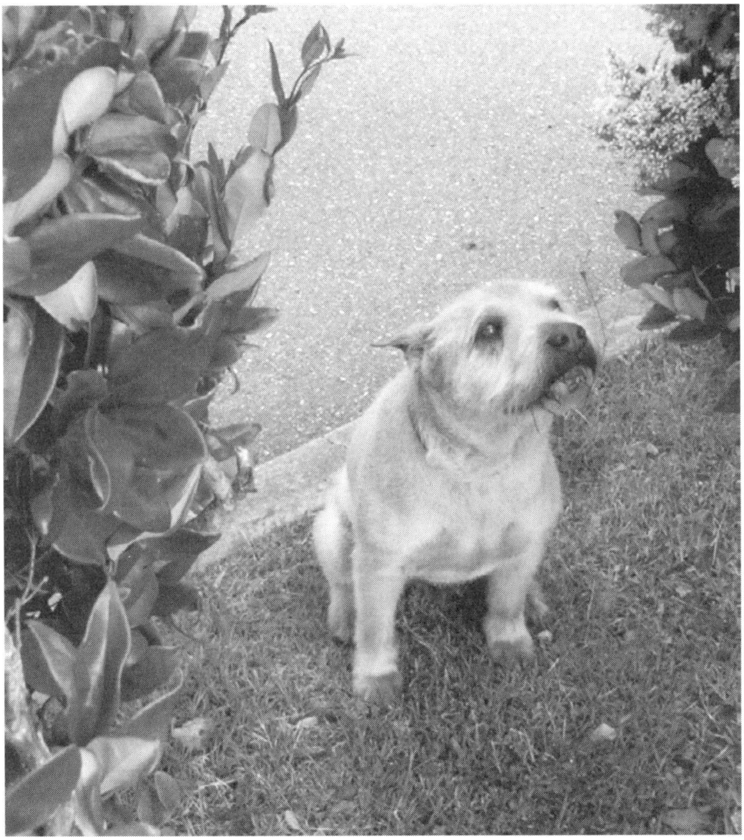

Photo 22

There are two other essential aspects of any exercise activity. They are *breathing* and *sleeping.* We avoided photos of these activities since neither is particularly photogenic.

Whether you're walking or doing one-arm handstands atop a 747's wing, no exercise will be of much benefit unless you *breathe*. Skeletal muscles in particular and the rest of the body in general are in constant need of oxygen. This is most important because exercises consume the most oxygen. Even our favorite pastime of sitting requires some oxygen to keep those unused muscles alive.

Andrew Weil, M.D. recognizes breathing as the single most vital activity in sustaining good health. We're not talking just breathing, which we all tend to do until dead. It's the *deep* breathing that really makes the beneficial difference. For too many urbanites, breathing barely keeps us alive since we don't work hard enough to do much heavy breathing.

Deep breathing—when you blow out (through your mouth) much of the air from your lungs, then suck as much air in (through your nose) as you can hold, plus another ounce. This does much more than prevent suffocation. Such deep breathing nourishes, cleanses and revitalizes your physiological functioning.

Dr. Weil's book, *Spontaneous Healing*, gives you worthwhile advice about healthful lifestyles, including deep breathing. His book is certainly worth reading. In the meantime, do a lot of deep breathing, especially when exercising and *never* when standing behind a running car or truck belching those exhaust toxins.

Equally indispensable to one's health and fitness is *sleep.* We all do it, but according to psychologist, James

B. Maas, Ph.D. the nation's leading sleep researcher, too many of us don't get enough of it. His research indicates that we, all of us, average 6.1 hours of sleep per night, while Dr. Maas has determined "we need 9.25 hours" nightly.

As important as the amount of sleep is the regularity of one's sleep schedule. Dr. Maas further explains that both the "sleep and wake schedule" and the amount of sleep are critical for good health. Relevant to this book, it's apparent that children and older seniors are especially affected by length or regularity of sleep. Dr. Maas's best selling book, *Power Sleep,* is another worthwhile read.

☙ ❧

Don't be alarmed. We have offered you enough excellent activities, aka exercises and their variations to keep you busy in any fitness club around the clock forever. You're certainly not expected to incorporate all of them into your revised lifestyle (except walking).

You don't need them all and you don't need a gym—unless it's really a social thing you need. If so, cut to the chase and join a social club. There are many in your area, they're less expensive than health clubs and with more undisguised social fun than any workout gym. As part of your new lifestyle, how about a dance club. They offer outstanding exercise and straightforward socializing. For the less budget cautious, tennis is a vigorous year-round activity with social spin-offs.

Golf is another socially promising, healthful activity, if you can afford it, forego the cart and *walk*. There are all sorts of people in your neighborhood who have been socially engaging in a healthy sport, like golf or tennis, as part of their way of life. They are your neighbors, so get to know them with an initial smile or wave.

More important, however, are those permanent changes in what you do or don't do every day—those activities that don't require schedules, meeting places or sitting. Like walking instead of driving (Photo 1), or a few morning and evening activities of your choice that may become part of your showering/tooth brushing routine. You can even burn a few more calories by hiding your remote control to facilitate getting up from your chair and walking to your TV to change the channel.

Some evenings, drop by your local library or bookstore. Wherever you go, either routinely walk or park a few blocks away. The change can become another regular activity. There are all sorts of health and fitness books waiting for you. You might find other exercises to easily combine with your new lifestyle activities. Yoga, for example, has numerous stretching and meditation routines that are appreciated by many people all their lives.

Since we're not selling a product or a service, we needn't reinvent the wheel. The only thing we have sold you is a book containing well-researched ideas. Putting these ideas into lifelong practice is free. So, as long as you find healthful activities and stick with them, your way of life will favorably change, along with your health and fitness.

Remember, even a loving dog provides a great addition to health and fitness lifestyle change. Aside from their loyal companionship, dogs love to take you for walks, be groomed, play Frisbee and any other healthful activity to remove you from your favorite TV-watching chair.

Here's another indispensable paradigm hinted earlier in this chapter. It's italicized because it's of value to anyone concerned with fitness and health. *Movement equals activity, which equals exercise.* Movement throughout our body is so essential to our well being, the absence of all movement is death to all of those muscles—even those we never knew were there.

Stop using the muscles for breathing and if the absence of oxygen doesn't kill you, lung congestion will. Simply lying in bed long enough without activity can easily cause blood clots (thrombosis). That's another way to die. Medicine finally figured out that minimizing movement by keeping patients in bed too long following an operation can be fatal. Non-movement interferes with the flow of blood, other tissue fluids, chemicals and oxygen's nourishment throughout the body. Even that muscle between our ears, the brain, demands those chemical movements (that perpetuate thinking, concentrating, etc.) or it dies.

And don't forget, activities are exercises that burn calories, reduce fat, build and tone skeletal muscles and make you healthier. That's provided they become your way of life and not just an occasional fad.

Clearly, the most effective time to develop a healthful lifestyle is at birth, before bad habits are established. So, in shaping behaviors, parents should be aware that, even for children, exercise is vital for health and fitness. An extensive scientific review by Journal of Pediatric Experts (2005) concludes that school-age children need *twice* the daily exercise/activities recommended for adults.

And flash, here's a no-brainer that the Surgeon General's office is finally acknowledging with long overdue clarity. The new food pyramid is emphasizing a common sense approach to good health and fitness called moderation in eating, plus exercising at least daily (or most days of the week). They add that activities such as "walking, dancing or gardening will cut your risk of early death."

Section M in the Appendix provides more vital information about the new food pyramid and your individual food and exercise regimen that clearly supports the strategy of this book.

☙ ❧

Here's a chapter closing anecdotal note of aching irony. A few weeks before this book went to press, our active Patti, who relishes walking, tripped over a dust-laden treadmill in her garage. She hit the concrete garage floor hard, causing sufficient injuries to prevent long, energetic walks for awhile. She also got rid of the treadmill.

Fact Summary

1. Movement equals activity, which equals exercise. So keep moving.
2. Walking is your most trustworthy health and fitness friend. Embrace it.
3. Every time you *move,* you burn calories.
4. Losing weight and flab doesn't require doing exercises "well" it simply requires doing more than before.
5. Any exercise apparatus you need in order to lose weight is available in your home.
6. This tip is for children who are old enough to crawl. Inform your parents (somehow) that kids need at least an hour's exercise/activity a day.

CHAPTER 14

If Your Menu's All Greasy, Toss It

Now that you have a more active lifestyle under your belt—so to speak, don't blow it on more food and bigger belts. The other half of your healthy lifestyle is every bit as important. It's time to focus on what and how much your eat!

Before you chow down, munch on our common sense menu. It's all about the obvious. Since eating is a necessary and fundamental part of all our lives, the question isn't to eat or not to eat. The questions are always what do we eat and how much. How much of our daily fuel (calories) intake do we burn? We have the freedom to eat *bad* and plenty of it, or learn how to eat *good* and less. Eating *good* requires some common sense and involves maintaining a healthy weight by eating sensibly, while enjoying what you eat.

Changing the unhealthy way you've been eating doesn't need to be a trial by ordeal. Anyway, that approach rarely works unless you're a masochist. We all eat either for *survival,* for *recreation*, to *compensate for life's dissatisfactions* or—for *no clear reason*. We all agree on the survival reason, we've got to eat to stay alive. What too many of us can't agree on is how much food we need to survive.

Here are your survival rules of thumb using equal activity rates. If you're overweight and gaining, you're not eating properly—probably too much. If you're slender, medically healthy and losing weight, you're not eating properly—probably not enough. For both problems, you need to reassess the type and amount of food you eat, and as boss of your matter, including your stomach, only you can change the way you eat.

If you're a recreational eater, chances are high that much of your social life involves eating. Besides, snack foods taste good. There are lots of restaurants and social get-togethers where eating and schmoozing flourish. How can we invite friends to our place without a tray full of fatty acid goodies? First step is to acknowledge that we consume twice the calories in restaurants than at home, and that most party snacks are no way to treat our friends. Then do something about it. Restaurants should be an occasional treat, not a constant habit. As for party snacks, there are low calorie, healthy ones. Many even taste good, and we don't mean just celery and carrot sticks.

If you're compulsively eating to compensate for feelings of depression, stress or some other disturbance, you have succumbed to a self-defeating behavior resulting in two problems for the price of one, and it simply doesn't work. If awareness of these symptoms doesn't help, see a therapist!

The most insidious reason for overeating may be the toughest to break. It's the "no clear reason" one, which is usually developing a habit of eating in a society that eats too much. Eating habits are a sneaky, complex result of the other three reasons for overeating. Remember, just eating as a habit puts your mind in *neutral*, with no thinking required. It's the *take-it-for-granted gear*. You just keep doing it over and over for no apparent reason other than everyone else is doing it.

For all of the above reasons for eating wrong, there's simply no way to eat right until you take charge of your mind to control your body. That's always the basic first step to behavior change. It also requires the courage and self-determination to think beyond those learned social boundaries.

For decades we took smoking for granted because of marketing and role modeling. Most everybody was doing it, including our favorite celebrities. Now researchers are telling us obesity is almost neck and neck with smoking as the cause of premature deaths in the United States. Get it?

ꟷ

It's time for step two, the transforming of good intentions into good eating habits—the other half of the health and fitness equation.

As you have probably figured out by now, there are all kinds of diets on the market insisting they're the best. Many are listed in the Bibliography section of this book, and each probably has merit, depending on your bankroll, common sense, resistance to quick fixes and a readiness for a lifestyle change. If you haven't done it already, look them over and you may find as I have that government diet recommendations make the most sense, especially if you're changing your lifestyle.

Accepting many of the American Medical Association (AMA), National Institute of Health (NIH) and Center for Disease Control (CDC) guidelines, my collaborating colleague and I have created a lifelong menu that thoroughly compliments the exercise half of our health and fitness equation. No, there's no magic to it, the menu just makes so much sense, I've been using it for years. It's a low fat menu that demands following a few easy fundamentals:

1. Don't take eating for granted. It leads to overeating and bad choices.

2. Avoid saturated fats, fatty acids and hydrogenated foods.
3. Choose the more healthful polyunsaturated and monounsaturated fats.
4. Reduce all fat intake to about 30% of your diet.
5. Read "Nutrition Facts" on any container of stuff you intend to eat. You'll be amazed.
6. Restaurant foods are loaded with tasty fats, salts and sugars.
7. Think *skull over crossed bones* when munching fatty meat.
8. If you're still working mainly at a desk, use your lunchtime to walk as you eat an apple.
9. Stay in charge of what you eat and you will live a longer, happier, more rewarding life.

No, I'm not a vegetarian and yes, I enjoy occasional meat, provided it's exceptionally *lean*. There are, however, some meats that deserve a warning label. Despite the generous three-page article "Going Whole Hog" in the San Francisco Chronicle (09/21/05), there are some meats I'll only nibble on once a year, or less. The meat is called "salumi" in Italian, which should mean tasty poison in English. Better known in the United States as salami, the ingredients include plenty of everything you don't need. It's a "curing" mixture of salt, sodium nitrate, live culture, sugar and flavorings. Trust me, you can really live without them—a lot longer.

As a septuagenarian in good health, I want to share with you my unabridged eating habits—in practicing what I've been preaching. Just about every morning begins with a glass of cranberry juice mixed with fiber and a few vitamin pills. Hardly an appetizer, that refresher is followed by about twelve ounces of fruit blended with a few ounces of apple, orange or cranberry juice. It is a delicious drink containing apples, bananas, pears, peaches, cantaloupe or a combination of any fruit in season. If you're losing teeth and like milkshakes, smoothies or tropical drinks without the booze, you'll love these. They're also pretty filling.

After reading a little of the newspaper, I have a big bowl of cereal, consisting of a variety of flakes, shreds, puffs and raisins. I buy the raisins separately because they're cheaper and Raisin Bran raisins in the box are like little pieces of gravel. Of course, I use non-fat milk, and I refrain from any cereal that even hints of *sweet*, like Cocoa Puffs, Frosty Flakes, etc. Pay no attention to the lure of those colorful cereal boxes. As usual, check the nutritional facts on the back of each box. That offers the real story about what you will be eating.

If I'm still hungry, which is rare, there's more cereal or whole wheat toast with jelly. I finish the paper with a strong cup of deeply black and delicious, fully-caffeinated, Columbian coffee—just one. No matter when I get up in the morning, I wait about an hour before eating for two reasons. Putting food in my mouth immediately after a night's sleep isn't appetizing, and a pre-breakfast walk with my dog for a few blocks clears my head, aerates my lungs and makes me hungry.

If you're a frugal shopper, this breakfast is remarkably inexpensive. There's generally some unpretentious cereal on sale, and produce market fruits are usually much cheaper than the major grocery chains. The cheap cranberry juice (made from concentrate) is also fine for me. Placebo or not, I haven't had a prostate problem in years. As for a blender, you can buy one at any of the big "Marts" for about $20. They won't pulverize rocks like the $600 models, which is okay, because I gave up eating rocks years ago.

Whistles blow, bells ring, courts adjourn, conferences stop, offices vacate, traffic swerves into rest stops and restaurants are ready. It's lunchtime folks! It's one of the most difficult habits to break and it has nothing to do with a biological need to eat. It does have plenty to do with a psychological response older than Pavlov's bell.

Our forefathers' twelve to fifteen hours of strenuous work a day is no longer necessary, but we still think we need their lunches. Well, as shocking as it may sound, we don't need lunches. We do need lunch breaks. The well-established excuse for lunch is our biological need for nourishment. Actually research in no way hints we'll be malnourished without lunch. Science does recognize, however, that a break in our daily work routine is a psychologically worthwhile stress reducer and a way to recharge our batteries.

Yes, kid's relentless growth and energy output requires a lunch of nourishing fuel—and I don't mean fries, burgers and Cokes. Hard working field hands and some construction workers, as well as some with medical problems may need noontime nourishment. For the rest of us, let's replace stuffing food in our face with resting, reading, socializing or even shopping.

Just about any work routine interruption, except eating, will enhance you health and fitness. If you must munch on something, grab some fresh fruit, like apples, pears, peaches, etc. They're all naturally sweet and good for you. Our matter is also just about always in demand of liquids, so drink plenty before, during and after lunch, and I don't mean martinis. Plenty of plain water is superb, followed by fruit juices, veggie juices and fruit concentrates. Even coffee and tea are included down the list, but not soda pop.

As for me, I don't eat lunch or "do lunch," and it's not because I wouldn't eat. It's because I would. I can eat at the drop of a hat, and it has nothing to do with hunger.

My dog is healthy, trim and so lovable he clearly communicates even though he can't speak in human tongue. When those big, brown button eyes stare up at me, I know what he wants—food. He stares up at me at least fifty times a day, and if I complied with his pleas, he'd look like a weather balloon and probably as helpless. After he has dinner and three biscuits, he acts as if he hasn't eaten in a month. My family and I know he would keep eating until he collapsed, and when revived he'd ask for more.

Well, I'm kind of like that, and I'm a human. Invite me over for a visit around noon and I'll most likely eat if you put a snack or plate of food in my lap. Potato chips? Since I can't eat just one, I can easily polish off a whole bag and not even know it happened. The point is, eating for we fortunates in our society has nothing to do with survival. We can eat anytime, anywhere and hunger is never a requirement. We seem to be constantly prepared to eat. We've learned the wrong cues well. Noon is time for lunch. Before the movie is time for popcorn and stuff. Sports events are times for hot dogs and stuff. At concerts, even the elite do intermission snacks and stuff. A social visit is a time for snacks and more stuff. And getting fat is becoming the sad rule, not the exception.

All of this has taught me that my dog and I don't need to eat ourselves to death. I've replaced much of the unnecessary eating activities with other more healthful ones. You can too.

Dinner for me is typically at around six p.m. because I'm ready for an enjoyable feast, followed by several hours of activities before going to bed at around eleven. Having a hearty meal is great. Just stay upright long enough to digest it.

What's for dinner? Turkey chili with a salad of avocados, tomatoes, onions, spinach, lettuce, asparagus, mushrooms, green olives, and any other veggies you like. Salad dressing is typically olive oil and Balsamic vinegar with a bunch of herbs and a ton of crushed garlic; some sourdough bread or tortillas to sop up the tasty juices, a glass of skim milk and another cup of 100% Columbian.

We have found that ground turkey has much less fat than ground red meat and its texture is so similar, people can't tell the difference—unless you wonder what happened to the grease.

Desserts are usually low fat pies and cakes, non-fat ice cream, yogurt or more chili if especially good that night.

Other entrée favorites are spaghetti with ground turkey, roast chicken, omelets, *lean* beef stroganoff, *lean* stews, *lean* meatloaf, tuna casseroles and plenty of boneless fish.

Entrees also include side dishes of steamed veggies, baked or mashed potatoes, and light gravies. Practically every night is salad night. I love salads, desserts and two cups of coffee a day—absolutely no lattés. In between the cups of coffee I drink green and black teas. During those warm afternoons in Arizona, I have a non-alcoholic beer, followed by a regular one—always moderation.

I, my family, colleagues and many of my friends are living demonstrations that you can be healthy and fit while eating virtually anything you want—as long as it's steeped in clear thinking, low fat, common sense and moderation, laced with activities. I can't vouch for your cooking, but I promise that with a little practice, your new menu will taste great and you'll feel even better about yourself.

☙ ❧

If you happen to feel a few twangs of bloat or heartburn after your healthful, sensible meal, don't despair. Second in importance to what you eat is *how you eat.* Whatever you eat involves a mechanical/chemical process of digestion; while indigestion, a too familiar word to all of us, is most commonly caused by eating like my beloved dog—too much, too fast.

Digestion prepares food for the final goal of absorption into such vitals as our blood. Here's roughly how it works. Next stop after the food reaches your fork, spoon or hand, it enters your mouth. Inside is the big receiving factory, the first step in digestion. There your taste buds, saliva and teeth go to work. The whole point is to break down your food from large pieces to smaller and smaller particles, until microscopically tiny.

Our teeth, real or false, are there to chomp, grind and crush food into small bits. The digestive enzymes in saliva mix with those food particles to further chemically prepare them for their digestive journey ending in absorption or elimination of whatever is left over through the bowels.

There's another important issue here. Without the taste buds toward the back of your tongue, everything would taste like dead tree bark and we would all really be skinny. Taste buds not only stimulate our eating, they help keep food in the mouth longer than one nano-second. If a mouthful tastes good, that food may linger long enough to break down by the mechanical/chemical mixing process. The longer it stays in your mouth, the less likely the bloat and heartburn.

So, don't take munching for granted. The only control we have over the process of eating is when the food is in our mouths. If we savor what's in there by eating slowly, another perk will be our increased enjoyment of the food with less need to stuff ourselves like my faithful dog does. In other words, slow down and you'll eat less, longer, enjoy it more and digest it better. Try putting your fork down after each bite.

These are lifestyle changes, not aerobics every Tuesday or another crash diet to try. Like kicking any bad habit, the first few months may be a bit awkward. If so, find a support group of people with similar lifestyles. There are plenty of them and unless you're a hermit, you'll definitely enjoy their company. Stay with your new lifestyle and you can't go wrong.

Fact Summary:

1. Take charge of your mind or marketing will do it for you.
2. A low fat, common sense menu of variety and moderation beats any special diet.
3. Unless you're "third world poor" you probably eat too much. Pay attention.
4. In "first world plenty" virtually every event you attend has unhealthy foods loaded with fat, sugar and salt. Be careful.
5. Learn how to read those "nutrition facts" on the back of labels. They're vital to your health.

6. It's not necessary to urgently change your lifestyle tomorrow morning. Just gradually keep changing it.
7. The next time you gorge yourself at lunch, ponder this unthinkable contrast. While the United States ranks as one of the first nations in world obesity, last place goes to those nations where 20,000 humans die of starvation daily.

CHAPTER 15

And the Winner is

As you enter our final chapter you may feel inspired, ready for change, even excited. Then again, you may be sensing a tinge of urgency or apprehension. Imagining changes in your life are fine, until you're faced with actually trying to change.

At last it boils down to *your* level of readiness to practice what *we* preach. It's your personal decision. Reading the book this far suggests you've learned a lot about your health and are motivated to change—unless you're one of those who, out of curiosity, begin at the end of books.

Even though it sounds great and seems worth a try, you may conjure up seven good reasons to put off trying until later. If that's the case, you're probably experiencing one of those "rationalizations" of the "all or nothing" challenge. You know, we've all been through it, like the salesman trying to intimidate you into buying that neat car you've been revisiting for weeks. It's the virtual moment of truth when, in so many words, the salesman barks a smiling "put up or shut up." Outwardly, your uneasy reply might be those seven "good" reasons for waiting. Inwardly, you're just not ready to invest in a new car—or to do all those healthful things. You're hardly ever *completely* ready.

Here's an important tip. If you are outwardly ready to permanently lose weight, to transform fat into muscle or just change a boring lifestyle of watching flab grow, try just a *little* change to begin with—no hurry, no deadlines, no contract and nothing to lose except excess weight.

Life isn't all or nothing, black or white, it's all about those fine nuances of gray. Unless you're into drowning, you don't learn how to swim by diving into the ocean. You splash around in the shallows as a first step. For you, that first step could be as subtle as a gentle walk around your neighborhood in the morning, evening or both. Actually, you've already started by simply knowing your health and fitness enemies and friends. You're probably already leery of those smooth talking enemies. That's a fine start in itself. Simply *not* taking your inactivity, lethargy and flab for granted invites change.

You'll hardly realize positive changes are happening—but they will. Here's an empirical example of dramatic and very positive changes in a friend of mine who had little interest in change and less in health programs.

Following the death of her husband, Sharon maintained a sluggish routine of cruise control inactivity. Drive to work, elevator to her office by 8:00 a.m., desk job until down the elevator at noon to soup and sandwich in the cafeteria. Then up the elevator, another four and a half hours of deskwork, and down the elevator to her car. Home by seven to a packaged, frozen food dinner, fall asleep on the couch watching TV, alarm blast at 5 a.m., shower and grooming, granola bars with coffee, out of the apartment into the identical routine, five days a week. Weekends were restaurant meals with friends, Saturday shopping, laundromat, video rentals, doze into couch sleep until 7 a.m. Sunday morning house cleaning, drive to church down the street, restaurant lunch with friends, home by 4 p.m., email, web-surfing, frozen lasagna with veggies, TV from couch, doze, sleepwalk to bed by twelve. At 5:00 a.m., weekday routine begins again. A very pretty lady, bulging with plump, she had been overweight most of her adult life.

Four years after her husband's death, Sharon met Frank, another old friend of mine. He's slender, healthy, active, but not fitness pushy. They would meet after work, and walk around her neighborhood before a real home cooked dinner he helped prepare. Sharon mentioned to me once that she had seen more of her city, San Francisco, with Frank than ever before. "Maybe," she added, "because for me the City was usually seen through a car window."

Frank and Sharon married a few years ago. Both in their upper sixties, they still stroll the City, holding hands, smiling at the sights and feeling rich. Sharon has no idea when, how or why she's thirty pounds lighter today.

"Gosh," she reasons, "I should be heavier, after all I'm older."

Frank doesn't know either. He didn't mind the plump. But *we* know, don't we? There was no fitness program, no diet regimen, no weight reducing deadlines—just a lifestyle change.

So, whether you're really ready or *kinda* ready, why not start with a neighborhood stroll. What are your neighbors up to? Are they friendly, reserved, stolid, grumpy, sleazy? Doesn't matter. Greet them all with a smile—it's your neighborhood. As explained earlier, eventually ninety-five percent will gratefully smile back. Even if they don't, smiling is contagious and, as you walk, you're burning calories.

Let those walks blossom into good habits. As you walk by, rather than into the Jack-in-the-Box, wave at the tall guy with the big round head. Then maybe have a piece of fruit during a lunch walk. It's a start, and you have a whole book of add-ons to your first steps. We promise you'll gradually loose weight, feel healthier, and you won't even know how it happened. And, whether it's two steps or two blocks more than yesterday's walk—the winner is you!

Fact Summary:

1. Avoid the "all or nothing" health challenge or you may end up with nothing.
2. Start all of your healthful lifestyle changes gradually.
3. The more active your lifestyle, the better your health and fitness.
4. The more enjoyable your lifestyle, the better your health and fitness.
5. The more sensible your eating habits, the better your health and fitness.
6. Health and fitness programs have high failure rates, while informed lifestyle changes don't.
7. As we grow older we need <u>more</u> not less exercise to keep ourselves trim.
8. Keep moving, stay active and greet your neighborhood with a smile. Don't forget, smiles also lead to calorie-burning laughs.

FOR SENIORS ONLY

Aging has its own way of telling us it's time to shift gears and start reinventing ourselves. The whispered message is to acquire a slower, more metered pace with thoughtful goals that match our rich past and sagging abilities. In terms of health and fitness, the worthwhile choices are endless. Here are just a few of the well documented ones we neglected to mention:

1. Caring for grandchildren, neighbors' children, anyone's children, will keep you more alert, active and trim.
2. Join or create a senior activity center in your neighborhood or community. There's a whole menu of activities you can offer, from walks with other seniors, neighborhood watch patrols, helping ailing seniors, to organizing First Aid courses and other classes by seniors with relevant skills.
3. Inexpensive trips to gambling casinos can be uplifting, calorie burning and socially gratifying, especially if you don't gamble.
4. Animal shelters always need dog walkers, and every city, town and village pleads for retirees to volunteer their skills to help others.

One of the tragedies of old age has nothing to do with not *being* needed—it's all about the delusion of not *feeling* needed.

Appendix

A. BODY MASS INDEX CHART

BMI (kg/m^2)	19	20	21	22	23	24	25	26	27	28	29	30	35	40
Height	Weight (lb.)													
4'10"	91	96	100	105	110	115	119	124	129	134	138	143	167	191
4'11"	94	99	104	109	114	119	124	128	133	138	143	148	173	198
5'0"	97	102	107	112	118	123	128	133	138	143	148	153	179	204
5'1"	100	106	111	116	122	127	132	137	143	148	153	158	185	211
5'2"	104	109	115	120	126	131	136	142	147	153	158	164	191	218
5'3"	107	113	118	124	130	135	141	146	152	158	163	169	197	225
5'4"	110	116	122	128	134	140	145	151	157	163	169	174	204	232
5'5"	114	120	126	132	138	144	150	156	162	168	174	180	210	240
5'6"	118	124	130	136	142	148	155	161	167	173	179	186	216	247
5'7"	121	127	134	140	146	153	159	166	172	178	185	191	223	255
5'8"	125	131	138	144	151	158	164	171	177	184	190	197	230	262
5'9"	128	135	142	149	155	162	169	176	182	189	196	203	236	270
5'10"	132	139	146	153	160	167	174	181	188	195	202	207	243	278
5'11"	136	143	150	157	165	172	179	186	193	200	208	215	250	286
6'0"	140	147	154	162	169	177	184	191	199	206	213	221	258	294
6'1"	144	151	159	166	174	182	189	197	204	212	219	227	265	302
6'2"	148	155	163	171	179	186	194	202	210	218	225	233	272	311
6'3"	152	160	168	176	184	192	200	208	216	224	232	240	279	319
6'4"	156	164	172	180	189	197	205	213	221	230	238	246	287	328

Risk of Associated Disease According to BMI and Waist Size

BMI		Waist less than or equal to 40 in. (men) or 35 in. (women)	Waist greater than 40 in. (men) or 35 in. (women
18.5 or less	Underweight	—	N/A
18.5 – 24.9	Normal	—	N/A
25.0 – 29.9	Overweight	Increased	High
30.0 – 34.9	Obese	High	Very High
35.0 – 39.9	Obese	Very High	Very High
40 or greater	Extremely Obese	Extremely High	Extremely High

B. BMI Formula using Meters and Kilograms

BMI = Kg/M²

1. Your height in inches times 2.54 = your height in centimeters.
2. Your weight in pounds times 0.45359 = your weight in kilograms.
3. Square your metric height.
4. Divide your kilogram weight by your squared height.
5. The quotient is your BMI.

BMI Interpretation

18 to 24 is healthy.
25 to 29 is overweight.
30 and higher is obese.
40 is morbidly (dangerously) obese.

Example: If you're 5′3″ and weigh 140 pounds, your BMI reads 25. That puts you in the overweight column—watch it.

C. Blood Pressure Basics

1. Sphygmonanometer is the gadget that takes your blood pressure.
2. The high number is called the systolic pressure when the heart is contracting.
3. The lower (smaller number) is called the diastolic pressure when the heart is relaxed between beats.
4. 120/80 or lower is good cardiac health.
5. 121 to 139/81 to 89 is pre-hypertension.

6. 140/90 if hypertension (high blood pressure).

Note: Lots of ailments are caused by hypertension.

Bottom line: Like the water pipes in your house, too much pressure and veins (pipes) can burst. The above numbers are just guidelines, so the lower the better.

D. **Pulse Basics**

The number of times your heart beats a minute is your pulse rate. The pulse in the wrist or carotid artery in the neck is easiest to find or feel. Use your index and middle finger pressure, not the thumb that has its own slight pulse. Normal pulse rate: 60 to 80 beats per minute, at rest.

E. **Type of Calories Per Gram**

Fat	9
Alcohol	7
Protein	4
Carbohydrates	4
Soluble Fiber	2

F. **Calorie Burning Activity Chart – Per Hour**

Walking at 2 mph	240 calories
Walking at 4 mph	440 calories
Jogging at 5.5 mph	740 calories
Bicycling at 6 mph	240 calories
Bicycling at 12 mph	410 calories
Swimming 25 yards/minute	275 calories
Swimming 50 yards/minute	500 calories
Tennis (Singles)	400 calories

Source: American Heart Association and National Heart, Lung and Blood Institute

G. **Stress Questionnaire**

Check the box below the scale from 1 to 5 that most nearly matches your agreement or disagreement with the statement as it applies to you. If you totally agree, mark the box under 5 and if you absolutely disagree, mark under 1. Mark box 3 if you can't decide.

		Totally Disagree 1	**2**	**3**	**4**	**Totally Agree 5**
1	My physical problems don't prevent exercising.	☐	☐	☐	☐	☐
2	I'm happy with the friends I have.	☐	☐	☐	☐	☐
3	Most of my friends stay in good shape.	☐	☐	☐	☐	☐
4	Controlling my temper is not a problem.	☐	☐	☐	☐	☐
5	I rarely get upset with my daily life.	☐	☐	☐	☐	☐
6	I'm very active during the day.	☐	☐	☐	☐	☐
7	I don't worry much about the life issues I can't control	☐	☐	☐	☐	☐
8	I have confidence in my coping abilities.	☐	☐	☐	☐	☐
9	I exercise regularly.	☐	☐	☐	☐	☐
10	Physically I'm in good shape.	☐	☐	☐	☐	☐
11	There's little stress in my life.	☐	☐	☐	☐	☐
12	Criticism from others doesn't bother me.	☐	☐	☐	☐	☐
13	I'm very satisfied with my life.	☐	☐	☐	☐	☐
14	I can always count on my friends for help.	☐	☐	☐	☐	☐
15	Trying to do my best is always good enough.	☐	☐	☐	☐	☐
16	I rarely get frustrated when things don't go my way.	☐	☐	☐	☐	☐
17	I have no chest pains or breathing problems.	☐	☐	☐	☐	☐
18	My mood isn't dependent upon the people around me.	☐	☐	☐	☐	☐
19	It doesn't bother me when I can't please everyone.	☐	☐	☐	☐	☐
20	My family and friends give me all the support I need.	☐	☐	☐	☐	☐
21	I avoid situations that might stress me out.	☐	☐	☐	☐	☐
22	My spirituality offers me peace.	☐	☐	☐	☐	☐

Scores	Lowest	Average	Highest
Stress Tolerance	22	66	110
Frustration Tolerance	10	30	50
Support Systems	4	12	20
Physical Health	5	15	25

H. Cholesterol Facts

Total Blood Cholesterol Levels

Less than 200 = ideal
More than 240 = high

Low Density Lipoprotein Levels (LDL)-Bad Cholesterol

Less than 100 = ideal
More than 160 = high

High Density Lipoprotein Levels (HDL)-Good Cholesterol healthy

Less than 40 = too low

I. Obesity Facts and References

- Obesity equals a BMI of 30 or above. Two-thirds of adults are overweight and people are getting fatter younger. Center for Disease Control and Prevention.
- Obesity at age twenty can reduce a person's life by twenty years. *Journal of American Medical Association (JAMA)*, January 8, 2003.
- Constant dieting efforts may be one central cause of depression in obese adults. Harvard School of Medicine, 2004.
- Obesity costs 93 billion dollars a year in health problems of the overweight. Center for Disease Control and Prevention in Atlanta, Georgia and RTI International.
- About 280,000 deaths a year are linked to obesity, including colon cancers in men, breast cancer and gall gladder cancer in women, plus gall stones, liver disease, osteoporosis and joint deterioration. *JAMA*, 1999, 282 (16) 1530-1538.
- Eating out significantly increases the number of calories you put away. Center for Science and Public Interest (CSPI) *Nutrition Action*, Page 12, U. S. Department of Agriculture.
- Ten Percent of pre-schoolers and fifteen percent of youth six to nineteen years of age in the United States are overweight. They all have a high risk for diabetes, asthma and high blood pressure before they

graduate from high school. All of them would greatly benefit from simple lifestyle changes. Robinson, Thomas, Stanford University, Lucile Packard Children's Hospital, *USA Weekend*, January 2, 2004.

- The better a person's fitness the better their physical and mental health, including self-confidence, self-image and self-control. Harvard School of Medicine, 2004.
- Salt increases the risk of hypertension, heart attacks, kidney disease and stomach cancer. Because of processed foods, we eat double the upper limits of salt. Eat low sodium foods. Institute of Medicine from *Readers Digest*, May 2004.
- Those people who drive rather than walk are significantly fatter. Redesigning cities to promote walking will help curb obesity. *American Journal of Health Promotion*, Volume 18, 1.
- We tend to eat more when given more. Packaged food products influence us to eat more. Having access to big portions of food can override our sense of fullness. *Nutrition Today*, Volume 38, 2, March/April, 2003.
- Overweight persons lose significant weight when in support groups, at least short term. Findings are mixed for long-term studies. Group treatment of weight loss is significantly better than individual therapy. *Monitor on Psychology*, Volume 35, 1, 56-58, January 2004.
- Even therapists, in treating obese clients, expect "less positive outcomes". *Obesity Research,* September 2003, Volume 11, 9.
- Overweight teenagers have fewer friends. Eating Disorders: *Journal of Treatment and Prevention*, Volume 8, 2, 2000.
- Fifteen percent drop in mortality of women eating eight servings or more of whole grains per week. Frozen foods are as good as fresh foods, sometimes even better. Health, How to Eat Smarter, *TIME Magazine,* October 20, 2003.

- Thirty minutes a day of moderate exercise, such as walking, led to fourteen pounds weight loss in one year, while much more vigorous exercise increased weight loss by only six more pounds. *JAMA*.
- People need fewer calories as they age. The formula is seven less calories a day for every year after age thirty for females and age ten for males. This means a thirty-one year old woman should eat 210 fewer calories a day than a thirty year old woman. Center for Sciences in the Public Interest, Nutrition Action, Volume 30, 7, September 2003.
- When a nationally syndicated newspaper headlines a message—it must be important. "Fatter Than Ever" was the San Francisco Chronicle headline on 08/25/05 taken from the California Center for Public Advocacy report a day earlier. The article says that despite all of the national alarm in the past several years about obesity in the United States, the BMI of kids in California has increased 6% since 2001. Researchers and politicians throughout the country agree that youth obesity isn't solely about school junk food and drink machines—it's about how "little exercise kids get."

J. <u>Activity Facts and References</u>

- "Exercise is the single most beneficial medicine in the nation." Exercise can control blood glucose levels in diabetics, prevent bone loss, reduce depression and reduce backaches. National Institute of Ageing, from *USA Weekend*, March 5, 2004, 13
- Walking at least four hours per week resulted in 40% less hip fractures than in those who walked less than an hour per week. A study of 6,000 women ages 40 – 72. Nutrition Action – Center for Science in the Public Interest. April, 2005, Volume 32, Number 3.
- People in the high risk group for cardiovascular disease, e.g. diabetics, smokers, those with hyper-tension and/or chest pains, are 45% less likely to die early with moderate exercise. Richardson, M.D., University of Michigan study.

- Consistent exercise (activities) five days per week significantly helps persons with Irritable Bowel Syndrome (IBS). Ted Mitchell, M.D., Wellness Program Medical Director, Cooper Clinic, Dallas, Texas.
- If you're overweight, keep moving. Any movements are better for your health and fitness than no movements. Science, 307, 530, 584, 2005

K. Body Composition

The percentage of fat in each individual, which differs from Body Mass Index, is determined by taking skin fold measurements at three body sites. For males the sites are: 1) a diagonal fold at the pectoralis muscle between the axilla and the nipple, 2) a horizontal fold at the umbilicus 5 centimeters from the navel and, 3) a vertical fold mid thigh between the patella and the hip joint. For females the sites are: 1) a vertical fold at the triceps at the back of the arm, 2) a diagonal fold at the iliac crest (top of the hip) and 3) a vertical fold at the front of the thigh, midway between the patella and the hip joint.

All measurements were taken at the subjects' right side as most studies are. These three site measurements are from a formula by Jackson and Pollock, leaders in the field of using skinfold measurements to determine body composition. Most authorities feel that skinfold measurements are a more accurate measure of determining the amount of "fat weight" a person has, rather than using the BMI formula, i.e. an athlete 69 inches tall with a body weight of 190 pounds will have a BMI of 28+, obese being 30. "However, the athlete, 69 inches tall and 190 pounds was a top decathlete," said Bob Lualhati, "who had only 8% fat."

L. Body Composition Standards

	Ideal	Overfat	Obese
Males	15-18%	19-24%	25%+
Females	20-24%	25-29%	30%+

M. **New Food Pyramid**

The United States Department of Agriculture (USDA) finally acknowledges individual differences in activity and dietary needs, and their new website provides required dietary food types and amounts based on your age, gender and activity rate.

Simply go to www.mypyramid.gov, answer a few basic questions and you'll have your personal dietary plan. If you're from the "quill pen" era, ask your grandkids for computer help.

N. **Solution to Child's Puzzle**

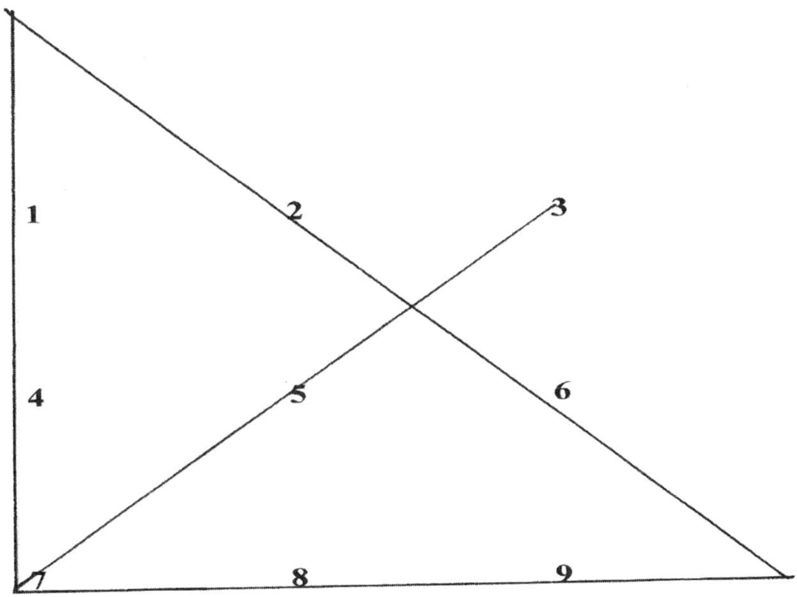

List of Photographs

Number and Activity	Page Number
Photo 1, Walking	114
Photo 2, Sitting without a chair	119
Photo 3, Push-up starting position	120
Photo 4, Full extended push-up	122
Photo 5, Modified full push-up	122
Photo 6, Sit-up starting position, down	123
Photo 7, Sit-up ending position, up	124
Photo 8, Bent leg sit-up	125
Photo 9, Leg-ups	125
Photo 10, Pelvis lift starting position	126
Photo 11, Pelvis lift extended	127
Photo 12, Flex Band starting position	129
Photo 13, Flex Band curl	131
Photo 14, Flex Band arm extension	133
Photo 15, Modified dip-up position	135
Photo 16, Modified dip-down position	135
Photo 17, Stair climbing	136
Photo 18, Stair climbing	137
Photo 19, Stair climbing	138
Photo 20, Shoveling	139
Photo 21, Dancing	140
Photo 22, Fitness Trainer	141

BIBLIOGRAPHY

Atkins, Robert C., *The Atkins Essentials*. Avon Books, 2004

Atkins, Robert C., *Health Revolution*. Bantum Books, 1990

Carper, Jean, *Stop Aging Now! The Ultimate Plan for Staying Young and Reversing the Aging Process*. Harper Collins, 1995.

Chopra, Deepak, *Perfect Health-Complete Mind Body Guide*. Three Rivers Press, 2000.

Chopra, Deepak, *Alternative Medicine*. Celestial Arts, 2002.

Conners, E, et al, *The Gold's Gym-Encyclopedia of Body Building*. Contemporary Books, 1998.

Edell, Dean, *Life, Liberty, and the Pursuit of Healthiness*. Harper Collins, 2004

Greene, Bob, *Get with the Program! Getting Real About your Weight, Health and Emotional Well Being*. Simon and Schuster, 2002.

Hastings, John, *The Breakthrough 12-Week Eating Plan. Change one-Lose Weight Simply, Safely, and Forever*. Readers Digest Association, 2004.

Jackowski, Ed J., *Hold It! You're Exercising Wrong,* A Fireside Book, Simon and Schuster.

Kalish, Susan, *Your Child's Fitness: Practical Advise for Parents.*

Karony, Stephenie and Ranken, Anthony, *Workouts with Weights*. Sterling Publishing Co., 1993.

Kirby, Jane, *Dieting for Dummies.* Wiley Publications, Inc., 2004

Kleiner, Susan, M. *Power Eating*. Human Kinetic, 2001.

Maas, Ph.D., James B., *Power Sleep.* Random House.

Markham, Douglas, J. *Beyond Atkins.* Total Health Care Publishing, 2004

McGraw, Phil, *The Ultimate Weight Solution. The 7 Keys to Weight Loss Freedom*. Free Press, 2003.

Packard, Andrew, *The Packard Weight Health Plan, Medically Based 5 Step Program for Permanent Weight Loss*, Ballantine Books, 2004

Perricone, Nicholas, *The Perricone Prescription*. Harper Resource, 2002

Phillips, Bill, *Body for Life, 12 Weeks to Mental and Physical Strength,* Harper Collins, 1999.

Rinzler, Carol Anne, *Weight Loss Kit for Dummies,* Hungry Minds, Inc., 2001

Tuttle, Dave, *Fifty Ways to Build Muscle Fast,* Avery, 2000

Weil, Andrew, *Natural Health, Natural Medicine – A Comprehensive Manuel for Wellness and Self-Care*, Houghton Mifflin Co., 1995

Weil, Andrew, *Eight Weeks to Optimum Health – A Proven Program for Taking Full Advantage of Your Body's Natural Healing Power,* The Ballantine Publishing Group, 1997.

Wennik, Roberta Schwartz, *Boomer's Guide to Getting the Weight Off – For Good,* Alpha Penigrin Group, 2003.

Wonderling, Lawrence, *SEDUCTIVE ILLUSIONS,* Cape Foundation, Inc., 1997

Articles

Allison, D., et al, *Annual Deaths Attributable to Obesity in the United States, Journal of the American Medical Association*, 1999, 282,16, 1530-1538.

DeAngelis, Tori, et al, *Battling Obesity.* American Psychological Association, *Monitor on Psychology*, January 2004.

Gerberding, Julie, Director, Center for Disease Control (CDC), *We're Eating Ourselves to Death.* Associated Press, March 9, 2004

Gorman, Christine, *How to Eat Smarter, TIME Magazine,* October 20, 2003.

Gupta, Sanja, *Fat Pill for Teens, TIME Magazine,* December 29, 2003.

Metropolitan Life Consumer Education Center, *Life Advise Pamphlet about Fitness and Exercise,* Metropolitan Life Insurance Company, 1996.

Mitchell, Ted, *So, You Wanna Know About Cholesterol?* Health Smart, *USA WEEKEND,* October 31 – November 2, 2003.

President's Council on Fitness and Sports, *Fitness Fundamentals.* Federal Government Consumer Information Catalog, Pueblo, CO 81009.

Preventing Obesity and Chronic Diseases Through Nutrition and Physical Activity, National Center for Chronic Disease Prevention, U. S. Department of Health and Human Services. September 24, 2003.

Robinson, Thomas, Associate Professor of Pediatrics, Stanford University, *National Association for Health and Fitness Newsletter. USA TODAY,* January 2, 2004.

Smith, Llene V., *Combating Obesity, NEWSWEEK,* March 22, 2004.

U.S. Department of Agriculture and U.S. Department of Health and Human Services, *Dietary Guidelines for Americans,* 2000

Wonderling, Lawrence V., *Rational Emotive Therapy in Central Asia, JOURNAL OF RATIONAL LIVING,* 9, 9-12.

INDEX

A
Activities, 90, 91, 142-146
Adaptability, 49
Adipose Tissue, xix, 6
Adipax, 23
Afghanistan, 46
AIDS, 31
Alcoholism, 59, 93
American Cancer Society, 13
American Medical Assn. (AMA), 59, 102, 144
American Psychological Assn. (APA), 14
American Society for Bariatric Surgery, 24
Anabolic Steroids, 108
Anatomy, 65
Antianxietants, 102
Antibiotics, 19, 20
Antidepressants, 102
Apparatus, 71
Aristotle, 34, 56
Atkins, 104
Attention Deficit Hyperactivity Disorder (ADHD), 34
All Terrain Vehicle (ATV), 115
Atrophy, 7, 72, 74, 117

B
Bariatric Surgery, 24, 101
Barnum, P.T., 56, 57, 70
Behavioral DNA, 62, 63
Bicycling, 114
Biochemical Programming, 15
Binge eating, 59
Biopsychosocial, 45
Blood Pressure, 58, 82, 85
Body Composition (BC), 28
Body Mass Index (BMI), 28, 29, 79-81, 118
Brain Behavior Relations, 45
Breathing, 142, 143
Burger King, 54
Bush, George W., 13

C
Calories, 55, 84, 114, 145 147 148
Cancers, 13, 14, 29
Caramelized, 57
Carmona, Richard, 14
Centers for Disease Control (CDC), 13, 24, 149
Cereals, 58-61, 151
Children, 116
Chopra, D., 104
Cognitive Behavioral Model, 94
Computerized Robotic Surgery, 18
Counselors, 102
Cruise Control, 90, 110-112, 159
Culture, 46
Curls, 129, 130

D
Dairy Queen, 54
Dancing, 65, 116, 140
Darwin, Charles, 7, 72
Depression, 93
Desoxyn, 23
Diets, 104, 105
Digestion, 155
Dips, 134, 135
DNA, 18, 62, 63, 78

Dogs, 118, 141, 151
Double Blinds, 107
Drug Problem, 64, 93, 94
DSM-IV, 34

E

Eating Habits, 147-150
Einstein, Albert, 25
Electric Carts & Chairs, 117
Empirical Data Collection, 106
Endocrine System, 44
Endorphins, 72
Enkephalins, 72
Enzymes, 23, 155
Excedrin Ads, 21

F

False Negatives & Positives, 84
Fat, xviii, 6, 16, 23, 24, 28, 35, 39, 46, 94
Faust, 34
Flex Bands, 127-134
First Aid, 19
Food & Drug Administration (FDA) 23
Food Group Pyramid, 21, 146
Fossil Fuel, 116

G

General Anxiety Disorder (GAD), 34
Genetic Code, 12
Genomes, 16, 18, 38, 46
Genotype, 11, 12, 16
Gollum's Ring, 44
Government Diet Recommendations, 149
Gupta, Sanjay, 23

H

Habits, 78, 112
Harvard School of Med., 167
Health Abuse Disorder (HAD), 34, 40
Health & Human Services Secretary, 13
Health Magazine, 70
Heredity, 12
HMO, 102
Homeostasis, 58
Homunculus, 74, 75
Human Genome Projects, 18
Hypertension, 13, 59

I

Immune System, 44, 103
Indigestion, 155
Inner Resources, 45
Intelligence Quotient (IQ), 16, 17

J

Jack-in-the-Box, 54, 67

K

Kline, Samuel, M.D., 24
Knowledge, 45

L

Liposuction, 24
Low Density Lipoprotein, (LDL), 53
Lualhati, Bob, xiii, 28, 29, 114
Lunch, 6, 7, 29, 152, 153

M

Maas, James B., Ph.D., 142, 143
Marketing, 7, 52, 53, 56, 58-61, 66, 68, 71, 74, 109
McDonald's, 54, 90
Medical Science, 18
Medications, 8, 93
Memory, 49
Metabolism, 16, 17, 24, 59

Methamphetamines, 23, 64
Millennium, Third, 4, 8
Mind, The, 39, 44, 87-97, 103, 110, 148
Mind Mirror, 89
Moderation, 34, 56, 156
Morphine Sulphate, 72
Movement, 145

N

Nat'l Academy of Sciences, 61
National Institute of Health (NIH), 149
Nervous System, 44
Neurobiochemical, 11, 64
Null Hypothesis, 107
Nutrition Facts, 150, 156

O

Obesity, xiv, 13, 14, 20, 23, 24, 32, 57, 93, 94, 149, 157
Orthopedic Physicians, 129
Over Fat (BC), 29, 170

P

Parallel Bars, 134
Parents, 26-28, 36, 37, 116
Pavlov, 6, 152
Peace Corps Trainees, 63
Penicillin, 19, 20
Perception, 92
Perricone, 104
Pharmaceutical Corp, 21, 22
Phenotype, 11
Physical Education, 30
Physical Therapists, 129
Physicians, 20, 21, 82, 83, 85, 102
Physicians Desk Reference, (PDR), 23
Pizza, 55-57
Population, World, 77
Polygraph, 45
Post Traumatic Stress Disorder (PTSD), 34
PPO, 102
Preventive Medicine (PM), 30-32
Prostate Problems, 85
PSA Test, 85
Psychiatrist, 62, 103
Psychological, 62, 103
Psychological Fingerprinting, 62, 90
Psychologist, 62, 103
Psychoneuroimmunology, 44
Psychotherapy, 37, 95
Push-ups, 120-122
Puzzle, 110, 111, 171

R

Rationalization, 49, 50
Readiness, 104
Reikian Body Work, 104
Religious Beliefs, 45
Rorschach, 89

S

Salt, 59, 94
Salumi (Salami), 150
School Exercise, 27
Schizophrenia, 33
Seadoos, 115
Septuagenarian, 150
Sex, 46
Simmons, Richard, 69
Sit-ups, 123
Skyline College, 28
Skeletal Muscles, 6
Sleep, 142-143
Smoking, 31, 149
Social Clubs, 143
Social Support, 45
Social Workers, 103

Spirituality, 45
Stairs, 71, 136-138
Steps, 70, 71
Streptococcus, 19
Stress, 92, 93, 102, 105
Stress Questionnaire, 94-96
Sugar, 59, 94
Sugarman, Harvey, M.D., 24
Surgeon General, 13, 145
Swimming, 65, 118
Syphilis, 19, 53

T

Technology, 66, 67
Theological, 51
Third Millennium, 4, 8
Thompson, T., 13
Thoughts, 44, 45, 48
Thrombosis, 145
Three R's, 26-28, 30
Time Magazine, 23
Treadmills, 69, 70, 146
Tuberculosis, 19
Tuttle, Dave, 104
Twenty First Century Paradox, 33, 67
Twenty Second Century, 74, 75
Twenty Values, 63, 91

U

United States Department of Agriculture (USDA), 171
Urban Society, 4, 35, 51, 105

V

Veterans Administration (VA), 102
Volition, 12, 16, 17

W

Walking, 73, 113-116,146
Water Activities, 118
Weil, Andrew, M.D., 104, 142
Wendy's, 54

X

Xenical, 23

Y

Yoga, 104,144

ABOUT THE AUTHOR

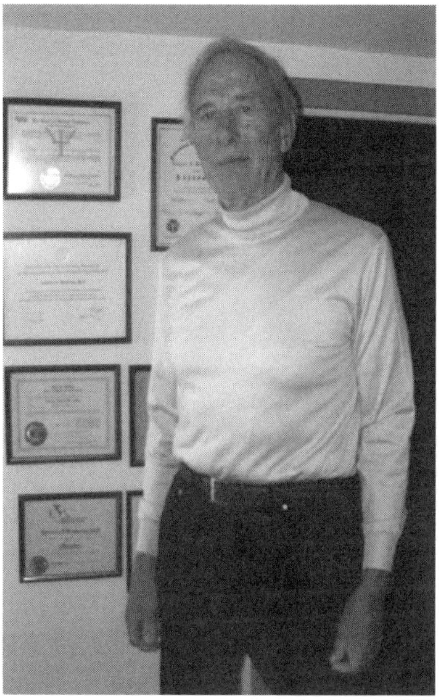

The clearest way to characterize Dr. Larry Wonderling is to describe his multifaceted background. Emerging from a poor, dysfunctional family he was a mediocre elementary school student who later earned a doctoral degree and the successful pursuit of three separate professions. He has been a clinical psychologist, an international cross-cultural consultant and is now an award-winning author. Athletically he achieved prep and college football Hall of Fame honors.

Today Dr. Wonderling is keenly aware that we're all capable of positive change, and that even obesity, along with associated suffering, is clearly preventable if we take responsibility for our lives and lifestyle. Practicing what he preaches, Larry Wonderling leads an active, trim and healthy life at the age of 75.